KV-683-994

A Better State of Health

John Willman is Consumer Industries Editor of the *Financial Times*.
He worked for many years for the Consumer's Association and wrote
several *Which?* books. Before joining the *Financial Times*, he was General
Secretary of the Fabian Society.

A Better State
of Health

JOHN WILLMAN

P
PROFILE BOOKS

First published in Great Britain in 1998 by Profile Books in association with the
Social Market Foundation

Profile Books Ltd
62 Queen Anne Street
London W1M 9LA

The Social Market Foundation
11 Tufton Street
London SW1P 3QB

Copyright © John Willman, 1998

Typeset in Bembo by MacGuru
macguru@pavilion.co.uk
Printed and bound in Great Britain by Biddles Ltd.

The moral right of the author has been asserted.

All rights reserved. Without limiting the rights under copyright reserved above,
no part of this publication may be reproduced, stored or introduced into a
retrieval system, or transmitted, in any form or by any means (electronic,
mechanical, photocopying, recording or otherwise), without the prior written
permission of both the copyright owner and the publisher of this book.

A CIP catalogue record for this book is available from the British Library.

ISBN 1 86197 089 7

Contents

Tables

Introduction

The National Health Service is one of Britain's great institutions which touches the lives of almost every citizen. The country's largest employer, it delivers us into the world, protects children from once-fatal illnesses, patches up those involved in accidents, maintains our bodies as parts wear out and helps us reach the allotted three score years and ten. And when the time comes for us to depart this world, it is often in the hands of the NHS that we make our exit.

Now – having reached the venerable age of 50 – the health service is itself ageing. And like many who reach their half century, time is beginning to take its toll. The world the NHS now finds itself in is very different from that of its youth, and the values it once espoused are being challenged.

One way in which Britain has changed – though people are often strangely loath to admit it – is that it is much wealthier. Per capita incomes have almost tripled during the lifetime of the NHS and many of the goods and services once beyond the reach of ordinary folk are now part of their everyday life. Yet for most of the health care we need, we continue to rely on a free state-provided service that rations out its limited resources using a variety of techniques from lengthy queues to simple denial of treatment.

The quality of the medicine practised in the British health service is probably as high as any in the world. But many of the institutions through which it is provided are shabby and variably organised to a degree that would be unacceptable in any other walk of life. And an honest observer would have to admit that the NHS has fallen behind the health services in other countries in terms of the treatment it offers and the quality of its service.

The commonplace assertion at this stage in the argument is that the NHS is underfunded, and that a modest increase in taxation could provide the resources it needs. Perhaps – though I suspect it would need a rather immodest tax rise, not just to meet the current funding shortfall but to raise the health service to the standards we might expect.

Although polls show voters clamouring to pay more tax to improve public services such as the NHS, the electorate has proved strangely reluctant to vote for parties that promise higher taxes. My own view is that for the last 20 years, people have become increasingly sceptical about whether higher taxes will produce better services. Once in the privacy of the voting booth, they prefer to hold on to their cash and vote against 'tax and spend parties'. Labour's election victory in 1997 was seen by some as the beginning of a new era. But the party's strategists believed – rightly, in my opinion – that their promise not to put up taxes was central to Labour's success.

In short, therefore, the contention of this book is that many – if not most – people would like to spend more on health services yet are unwilling to do so through a state-financed National Health Service. The question it seeks to answer is how they can be allowed to spend more of their own money on health care without leaving those who cannot afford to pay more relying on some sort of second-class, state-funded safety net.

This book also argues that the quality of health services would be improved if people made a direct contribution towards them. A state-financed service that provides free health care treats all patients as having identical needs and thus ignores their individual requirements. If people were paying they would demand – and get – better quality services tailored to their particular circumstances, and to a standard comparable with the best private sector services.

Finally, it suggests that one of the commonest arguments for maintaining a health service free at the point of use bears closer examination. Most other countries have some form of charging for health care, and many have much less inequality in the health of their citizens. While a free NHS in theory removes a barrier to access, in practice those it aims to benefit fail to take advantage of what it offers. Charging those who can afford to pay might provide resources which could be used for a concerted attack on health inequalities.

To say such things will be seen by many as impertinent – an act of great ingratitude. As a child of the post-war welfare state, I clearly owe a debt to an institution which brought me into the world, protected me from childhood diseases, extracted my appendix – and now does much the same for my children. As the son of a doctor – and the son-in-law of another – I have also benefited personally from the noble profession of medicine.

Many inside and outside the health service will be angry at my presumption – and even more enraged by this book's conclusions. How could a mere journalist dare to challenge a pillar of British society in which more than a million dedicated people strive to cure illness and alleviate suffering?

To borrow a phrase from the 1997 Labour general election campaign, Britain deserves better – a health service that provides the health care people want. There are many obstacles to creating such a service, not least the ingrained belief that the NHS is the best in the world or that the only alternative is an American-type system that bankrupts patients and leaves millions without cover. Yet in most western countries, health services are available to all without long waiting lists or other objectionable forms of rationing – and without creating unacceptable costs.

This book is an attempt to see how Britain could enjoy a similar standard of health care. I hope readers will accept it is not written as a wanton ideological assault on the NHS, which has served the British people well. Rather it is an attempt to examine how it measures up to its ambitions and, when it fails to achieve them, identify the reasons.

For those who like simple and revolutionary solutions to such problems, the conclusions will be a disappointment. There is no sweeping change proposed – no wholesale switch to private insurance or any other magic pill. I have tried to sketch out a feasible way forward that allows people to contribute more to their health care while preserving much of the NHS. A system that aspires to provide health care for all must find some way of sharing out the cost of dealing with the accidents, emergencies and seriously life-threatening illnesses which no commercial insurance system will cover without excessive regulation. The health service is as good a system as any for doing that, though some ways to pep it up are suggested in the final chapter.

Even this relatively modest blueprint will, however, prove

contentious. There are many vested interests that can be relied upon to shout loudly against any change in the health service. Chief among these is the British Medical Association which opposed the creation of the NHS and has fought almost every change to the original design ever since. The vast majority of patients, health workers – even doctors – might benefit from changes to raise standards in the health service, but there are no powerful lobbies arguing for change and the public is rightly sceptical of anything politicians might propose.

I ask only that readers judge the book's argument with an open mind and think deeply about the issues raised. There are important questions about the sort of society Britain is and the way it helps the people who benefit least from the present health care arrangements. Those opposed to change all too often paint critics of the NHS as ideologues bent on wrecking a great national institution. But turning the health service into what one analyst has described as 'Britain's only immaculate institution' does no one any favours. [1]

There are many debts in writing such a book. One of the greatest is to the legion of researchers and health service professionals who have provided me with its raw material. Many – if not most – will disagree with the conclusions to some degree or other. Quite a few may feel outraged where I have lifted their thoughts and theories, in some cases in great detail.

My contribution as a journalist is to do what I earn my living from: assembling diverse facts and opinions, binding them together in an attempt to give new insights and writing the product in as accessible a form as possible. I have tried to give sources throughout, but no one should assume that any researcher credited has any sympathy with the book's argument.

Two other important debts are to the *Financial Times* and the Social Market Foundation. I joined the *FT* in 1991 as Public Policy Editor, observing at close hand the introduction of the Conservative health reforms and the ensuing struggles. With the advantage of working for an international newspaper, I was able to report the changes in the NHS from a perspective informed by what was going on in other countries.

It threw a rather different light on the British changes, as part of a global struggle to modernise health services and update welfare provisions devised decades earlier. I am deeply grateful to the *FT* for the opportunity and even more to its enlightened policy of granting all its journalists sabbaticals to allow time to analyse and write in depth.

In my case, the Social Market Foundation offered the framework to develop the analysis, in the form of a Gatsby Visiting Research Fellowship during the summer of 1997. It was only the rugged persistence of Roderick Nye, the SMF Director, that persuaded me of the wisdom of contemplating such a project. I am grateful to him and to all of the SMF staff for their ideas, support and friendship – a debt that extends also to Lord Skidelsky, the Foundation's distinguished chairman.

Special thanks are due to Jessica Barrington, then a research officer at the SMF, for tracking down various documents and in drafting parts of Chapter 8. She also organised two seminars at which aspects of the argument in this book were tested. Helen Brown organised a third.

My thanks to all those who attended those seminars, but especially to the two who presented papers: Julian Le Grand, Richard Titmuss Professor of Health Economics at the London School of Economics; and Deborah Baker, Senior Research Fellow at the Department of Child Health, Bristol University. Valuable comments on the first draft were received from Rifat Atun, Mark Bassett, Nick Bosanquet, Tony Hockley and Alastair Kilmarnock. None of these individuals is responsible for errors in the text or faults in the argument – but there are fewer of either as a result of their efforts.

I am grateful to the staff in the libraries at the *FT* and at the King's Fund – the latter an asset of incomparable worth for those interested in health policy. Anyone who studies the economics of health care is also indebted to Jean-Pierre Poullier of the Organisation for Economic Co-operation and Development: he has built up an indispensable database of health statistics which allows sensible cross-country comparisons to be made.

The final product owes much to Andrew Franklin, Stephen Brough and Nicky White at Profile Books.

1: A Health Service to be Proud of?

Ask a random sample of people to rank a series of institutions in Britain and chances are the National Health Service will come out well. Support for traditional pillars of British society such as the monarchy, Parliament, the church and the legal system may be plummeting. But the NHS general practitioner came out top in a list of trusted institutions and consumer brands in a poll carried out by the Henley Centre, the market research organisation.[1]

The health service's 50th anniversary on 5 July 1998 will be marked by celebrations throughout the UK that will recall its noble beginnings and great achievements. Tony Blair has already set the tone in his foreword to a history of the first half-century published by the King's Fund, the health care think-tank. He describes the NHS as an institution that has changed the lives of generations of men, women and children:

> Major advances in science, technology and information give us access to treatments and therapies today which would be unrecognisable to the architects of the National Health Service in 1948. However, amidst all the advances, the founding principles upon which they built the NHS have stood firm, providing a quality service for all, regardless of ability to pay.[2]

But is the National Health Service all that it is cracked up to be? Comparing its performance with other countries' health services indicates some disturbing shortcomings. And a series of reports from various watchdogs suggests the NHS could perform much better – both medically and in the stewardship of its funds. We begin, therefore, by looking in more detail at the popularity of the health service – and ask whether it is deserved.

The people's choice

The most consistent picture of the state of UK public opinion on the public services is provided by the British Social Attitudes survey. Since its first poll in 1983, it has asked the same questions about priorities for public spending and people's willingness to pay extra tax for better services.[3]

Each year for example, it asks how satisfied people are with 'the way in which the National Health Service runs nowadays'. Table 1.1 shows the results over the years.

Table 1.1
Satisfaction with the NHS

	1983 %	1986 %	1990 %	1993 %	1996 %
Satisfied	55	40	37	44	36
Not satisfied or dissatisfied	20	19	15	18	14
Dissatisfied	25	40	47	38	50

Source: Ken Judge, Jo-Ann Mulligan and Bill New, 'The NHS: New prescriptions Needed?' in Roger Jowell et al (eds.), *British Social Attitudes – The 14th Report*, 1997, p. 53.

Thus levels of dissatisfaction have doubled in recent years, with half those asked being unhappy with the NHS. When the British Social Attitudes survey started, the majority was satisfied, outnumbering the dissatisfied by two to one. Today barely a third are satisfied, despite an upturn in satisfaction in the early 1990s after the Conservatives' 1991 NHS reforms.

Throughout the period of the survey, there has been a consistent demand for more spending on health care. Even in 1983 when more than half those asked said they were satisfied, almost two-thirds still wanted more spent on the NHS when asked to name their two highest priorities for extra public spending. As Table 1.2 shows, health has remained the top priority throughout, with more than three-quarters now supporting extra spending.

Table 1.2
Spending priorities

Support for extra spending on	1983	1987	1991	1995
	%	%	%	%
Health	63	78	74	77
Education	50	55	62	66
Defence	8	4	4	3
Help for industry	29	11	10	9

Source: Lindsay Brook, John Hall and Ian Preston, 'Public Spending and Taxation' in Roger Jowell et al (eds.), *British Social Attitudes – The 13th Report*, 1996, p. 186.

The British Social Attitudes survey also tries to establish people's willingness to pay for increases in spending on health, education and social benefits. As Table 1.3 indicates, the majority view has shifted on this since 1983.

In the first year of the survey, most people wanted to keep

taxes and spending on these services the same, with less than a third prepared to pay extra taxes to boost spending. Since then, support for higher taxes has risen, and now outnumbers those happy with the status quo by two to one. Tax-cutters have diminished in number, with only one in twenty wanting lower taxes and less spending on health, education and social benefits.

Table 1.3
Preferences for tax and spending on health, education and social benefits

	1983 %	1987 %	1991 %	1995 %
Increased taxes and more spending	32	50	65	61
Keeping taxes and spending same as now	54	42	29	31
Reducing taxes with less spending	9	3	3	5

Source: Brook, Hall and Preston, 1996, p. 187.

Support for higher spending on health and other public services thus falls somewhat if an increase in taxes is needed to pay for it. But the survey shows a comfortable majority now favours such higher spending nonetheless – support that is consistent across income groups, the sexes and age groups. The survey also gives an indication of why there is this growing demand for extra spending. The proportion of people who are satisfied with the NHS has fallen since 1983 – as Table 1.4 shows. Satisfaction is least among younger age groups and professionals – the next generation of voters and those at the top of the social ladder.

Table 1.4
Satisfaction with the NHS

	% satisfied		
	1983	*1989*	*1993*
All	55	37	44
Men			
18–34	45	27	32
35–54	51	31	39
55+	61	46	54
Women			
18–34	55	33	36
35–54	52	36	44
55+	61	46	58
Social class			
I – Professional	52	36	38
II – Managerial	52	38	47
III – Non-manual	54	36	45
IV – Manual	59	37	44

Source: Nick Bosanquet and Anna Zarzecka, 'Attitudes to Health
Services 1983 to 1993', in Anthony Harrison (ed.), *Healthcare UK
1994/95*, 1995, p. 89.

This level of dissatisfaction is confirmed by a 1996 Eurobarometer survey on health services in 15 EU countries spon-
sored by the European Union.[4] It found 48.1 per cent of
those questioned in the UK were fairly or very satisfied with
the NHS – not far off the EU average.

Table 1.5
Satisfaction with health services in the EU, 1996

	% satisfied	Health spending per head, 1995, $*
Germany	66	2,134
France	65	1,956
Netherlands	73	1,728
Belgium	70	1,665
Austria	63	1,634
Italy	16	1,507
Denmark	90	1,368
Sweden	67	1,360
Finland	86	1,373
UK	**48**	**1,246**
Ireland	50	1,106
Spain	36	1,075
Portugal	20	1,035
Greece	17	703
EU (15)	50	

* In $, converted at purchasing power parities – see p. 169.
Source: Elias Mossialos, 'Citizens' Views on Healthcare Systems in the 15
Member States of the European Union', *Health Economics*, vol. 6, 1997,
p. 111; purchasing power parities from BMA, *Options for Funding
Healthcare*, 1997, p. 4.

However, the comparison with other EU countries throws
up an interesting result. By and large, satisfaction ratings in
different EU countries reflect spending per head on health
services – Italy being a conspicuous exception. But three
other countries in the middle of the spending league table

with the UK – Sweden, Finland and Denmark – record much greater satisfaction with their health services.

Another question in the Eurobarometer survey indicated rather deeper dissatisfaction with the health service in the UK than in other countries. The question asked whether reforms were needed in the various countries' health care systems. In the UK, just 14.6 per cent thought that the NHS ran 'quite well' on the whole, with 27.4 per cent thinking minor changes were needed. But 42 per cent thought fundamental changes were needed and 14 per cent that the NHS required complete restructuring. Only Italy, Greece and Portugal had larger proportions thinking fundamental reforms were needed.

As in the British Social Attitudes survey, Eurobarometer found a high level of demand for extra spending on health in the UK – at 81.5 per cent, it was second only to Greece in the proportion wanting more. The average for the 15 EU states was 48 per cent. But unlike British Social Attitudes, the Eurobarometer survey found only 28.8 per cent of the UK sample wanted higher taxes to pay for more spending. This was perhaps because they were offered another option of finding cuts in other budgets to pay for higher health spending – an option most chose.

What can we learn from this conflicting evidence? First, whatever people say about the NHS being the best in the world, there is great dissatisfaction with it. Second, most people expect the government to spend more to bring it up to scratch. But third, there is contradictory evidence of their willingness to pay for increases in spending through higher taxes. Whatever people say in the British Social Attitudes survey, they have proved remarkably unwilling to translate support for higher taxes into votes for parties prepared to raise them in successive general elections.

The best health service in the world?

But is the public right to be dissatisfied with the National Health Service? With life-and-death emergencies, the NHS appears to be up with the best internationally. A patient in need of a bone marrow transplant is as likely to have the operation in the UK as in the US.

However the UK falls behind other countries in routine surgery and high-technology care. For example, Britain devotes much less resources to relieving pain – the Americans perform 10 times as much coronary heart surgery.[5] And a report covering south-west London and other parts of the south-east suggested that hospital mortality rates for those in intensive care were 25 per cent higher than would be expected for a similar group of American patients: the equivalent of some 240 deaths a year.[6]

Kidney dialysis is another example where the UK falls behind other countries. This is an acknowledged life-saving form of treatment but one that is also expensive. Since its introduction in the 1960s, it has been rationed in the National Health Service by a variety of means. First it was restricted to regional centres as a new technology needing specialised resources. Later it was effectively withheld from older patients and those with other medical complications.

The rationing of kidney dialysis treatment by withholding it from older patients was described in the 1980s by two American researchers:

Confronted by a person older than the prevailing
unofficial age of cut-off for dialysis, the British GP tells
the victim of chronic renal failure or his family that
nothing can be done except to make the patient as
comfortable as possible in the time remaining. The
British nephrologist tells the family of a patient who is
difficult to handle that dialysis would be painful and
burdensome and that the patient would be more
comfortable without it.[7]

The UK treats significantly fewer patients with renal failure than the European mean – and the gap is widening.[8]
Britain ranks 21st in Europe in the number of new patients
treated each year, according to the European Dialysis and
Transplant Association. Only Bulgaria treats fewer patients
per head of population per year.[9] The founding vision of the
NHS was of a comprehensive health service available to all
free at the point of use. But when it comes to kidney dialysis, you are more likely to get it in America where it has to be
paid for.

This observation should not be seen as an endorsement of
the American health care system which has problems far
more serious than anything facing the NHS. Both systems ration health care: in Britain, all are eligible but must stand in
queues; in America, few wait for treatment but some are left
out altogether. However, the acknowledged failings of the
American health care system – which are entirely predictable
in any system that relies entirely on private insurance –
should not blind us to the shortcomings of the British
model.

Kidney dialysis is perhaps an extreme example of the way the NHS rations treatment. But the same is true with other expensive forms of treatment. For example, the shortage of lithotripters which use shockwaves to disintegrate kidney stones without surgery means this technique is much less common than in many other European countries. The UK has one lithotripter for every 3.8 million people, compared with one for every 800,000 in Belgium.[10]

Even within the UK, there are enormous variations in the treatment available in different parts of the country. Table 1.6 shows the variations between health authorities for five common procedures.

Table 1.6
The treatment lottery

Procedure	Rates of treatment per 100,000 residents			
	Min. rate	Max. rate	Bottom 10%	Top 10%
Cataract surgery	149	469	201	363
Coronary artery bypass graft	0.5	59	5	42
Hip replacement	36	152	51	110
Knee replacement	18	86	29	64
Tonsillectomy	8	403	102	263

Source: Department of Health, *Health Service Indicators 1993–94*, in Rudolf Klein et al, *Managing Scarcity*, 1996, p. 670.

The figures in Table 1.6 make no allowance for the different needs of the people covered by the various health authorities. But even allowing for that, they show variations in the levels of treatment within the NHS that can have little to do with need. With cataract surgery, for example, the district treating the highest proportion of its population is carrying out three times as many operations a year as the district performing the least. In some cases there may be fluke figures at the top or bottom of a range, but comparing the average for the top 10 per cent of health authorities with the lowest 10 per cent indicates similar variation. For example, you are more than eight times as likely to have a coronary artery by-pass graft in the top 10 per cent as in the bottom 10 per cent.

Far from delivering a universal health service, free at the point of use, the NHS provides a greatly varied service in different parts of the country. And in access to some forms of treatment, the NHS falls far behind other countries.

Hospitals – full of sick people

Nor is getting into hospital a guarantee of good treatment. Some 100,000 people a year – 10 per cent of patients – contract an infection while in hospital, according to a study by the Office of Health Economics.[11] Infections contracted while in hospital cause 5,000 deaths a year and contribute to a further 15,000, making them a bigger killer than road accidents.

The delays in recovery as a result of hospital-acquired infection cost hospitals up to £3,600 per patient in extra medicine and longer stays. Overall, the cost to the NHS is more than £170 million a year – and while these infections cannot be eliminated, according to the study they could be cut by up to a third. In America, hospitals employ one nurse to control hospital acquired infections for every 250 beds but in the UK, there is only one for every 477 beds.

The rate of infection is not helped by the decrepit state of many NHS hospitals, which are still housed in 19th century buildings – some designed as workhouses. But even in modern hospitals in the leafy suburbs, conditions are far from ideal for sick people. One patient who was admitted for a simple toe-straightening operation discharged herself on the second day after finding the following:[12]

- overflowing ashtrays in a no-smoking day room
- dirty wards (a cleaner said 'You could grow potatoes under there', when the patient pointed out dirt and fluff under her bed)
- crowding in mixed-sex wards – 'the beds were so close you could reach across and touch your neighbour'
- poor quality meals – using the system common in many hospitals, meals were ordered a day in advance, so the first day's meals had usually been ordered by the person discharged the day before
- shortage of simple equipment such as a cradle to support bedclothes and a wheelchair.

The trust that ran the hospital had various mission statements and placards announcing its wish to deliver the highest quality care. But the gap between the rhetoric and the reality could not be blamed on a shortage of resources, according to the patient – the place was simply badly managed. She should know: a former NHS employee, she is now a researcher on health and clinical services management.

Hospital catering is a recurrent complaint among patients. A 1997 study of four general hospitals found meals often arrived late and poorly presented. The NHS spends more than £500 million a year on hospital catering, making it the third largest purchaser of catering services in the country. But the study calculated that almost half the food served is thrown away – not only a waste of money but a failure to meet the needs of patients recovering from treatment.[13]

The astonishing thing is that people put up with such conditions – largely because they have such low expectations of the NHS. A 1997 *Which?* report on hospital stays compiled a long list of complaints from a sample of 30 recent hospital patients.[14] Two had had to wait longer than 18 months for admission to hospital, while eight had had their first hospital admission dates cancelled – in one case with a delay for a further 10 months. Once in hospital, several were unhappy about the lack of privacy in wards – particularly mixed-sex wards. Others felt abandoned after being shown to their beds, or were given too little information. One reason they didn't always ask the questions they wanted to was their reluctance to make demands on nurses who appeared 'stressed' and 'overworked'. The lack of privacy on wards also inhibited them from asking for information.

Despite such criticisms, the patients were 'generally happy with the care and attention they received and impressed with hospital facilities'. This was because they perceived the NHS to be 'run on a shoestring' with staff and bed shortages, long waiting lists and antiquated hospitals. As a result, most were 'pleasantly surprised that their stay in hospital turned out to be better than they had expected'.

Few would tolerate these conditions on holiday or on a business trip when they had paid for the accommodation.

Imagine your reaction if your package holiday turned out to involve sharing a mixed ward dormitory. Or if the staff in a hotel were so stressed and overworked that you could not get the service you were entitled to. Yet these conditions are accepted as normal when we undergo the far more stressful experience of hospital treatment.

A question of money?

The shortage of resources is certainly responsible for some of these problems – it would cost more for every patient to have a room of their own, for example. But there is a more fundamental shortcoming that reflects the ethos of a service provided free to all as a gift of the state. This plays down the patient's needs – whether they are privacy, decent food, prompt appointments or tolerable delays in waiting for operations. It also leads many NHS institutions to ignore the practices of normal commercial life and waste scarce resources in ways that would appal patients if they knew about it.

One good example is the way hospitals and other NHS organisations waste around £50 million a year on radiological services – X-rays, ultrasound scanning and magnetic resonance imaging. These techniques are invaluable in diagnosing patients and monitoring their treatment – and cost the health service £600 million a year. But a study by the Audit Commission, the public spending watchdog, found some radiology departments spent nearly twice as much as others with a similar workload. If all hospitals adopted basic procedures in deciding when these expensive techniques should be used, the Commission calculated the health service could save some £30 million a year.[15] The Audit Commission report also says a fifth of X-ray examinations are unlikely to help patients and may involve radiation risks. At one hospital, three-quarters of chest X-rays taken before operations were never even taken out of the packet for examination. Savings of £24 million could be made by cutting these out.[16]

Similar waste was found in hospital spending on supplies such as medical and surgical equipment, building materials, printing and stationery. These cost the NHS £4.4 billion a year, but some acute hospitals spend 50 per cent more on clinical supplies than others with a similar mix of patients and treatments, according to another report from the Audit Commission.[17] For example, trusts were paying between £825 and £1,420 for identical models of the syringe drivers used to administer steady amounts of drugs.[18]

The report concluded that some simple improvements in purchasing methods and stockholding could save £200 million over a three-year period. For example, one small acute hospital trust could have saved £6,900 (17 per cent) of the £39,600 annual cost of buying rubber gloves if it had bought only the cheapest of the six brands it was purchasing.[19] Another could have saved £8,000 a year if it had bought all its syringe drivers at the price paid by two wards which purchased them for less than £800 – two others were paying more than £1,000 for the same model. Overall, the trust might have been able to make even greater savings by placing a single order to get the maximum discount. (Interestingly, the highest price was paid by wards which had been given extra funds to cut waiting lists and for other developments. Extra money is no guarantee of a solution to the NHS's problems.)

Purchasing methods often wilfully neglect good value for money, according to the Commission. The cost of placing orders for about a quarter of the purchases made by the 15 trusts it visited was greater than the price of the goods.[20] And hospitals could save £7 million a year by paying bills on time – many suppliers offer discounts if payment is received within 30 days. Some trusts pay bills late to manage cash flow (which is against government policy) – but more often the cause is 'poor systems design or over-cautious payment procedures', the Commission says.[21]

There is also wastage in the amount of stock hospitals are holding. Some provincial acute trusts hold more than £30,000 of stock for every £1 million they spend, while others get by with less than £10,000.[22] Excess stock ends up passing its use-by dates, becomes obsolescent or is a target for pilfering. The Commission estimated computerised stock-holding could reduce the cost of NHS stores by £50 million in England and Wales.

Such sloppy practice wastes money, but it also poses a threat to patients. If hospitals end up with a wide variety of equipment, staff could find some of it unfamiliar. One of the trusts visited for the Audit Commission study, for example, had 30 different models of syringe driver while another got by with 13 models.

Supplies account for between a fifth and a quarter of the money spent by trusts. But, according to the Audit Commission, most senior managers have shown little interest in their cost. The Commission found that only five of fifteen trusts visited had discussed supplies at board level. Executive directors responsible for supplies estimated they spent no more than 5 per cent of their time on supplies matters.[23]

Hospital managers and doctors complain of a shortage of resources and explain shortcomings as a consequence of government parsimony. But Audit Commission reports indicate a systemic failure of hospitals to husband the resources they have.

Accident and Emergency treatment

The performance of Accident and Emergency (A&E) departments illustrates the failure of the NHS to put the patient first. Every year, 15 million visits are made to A&E departments in England and Wales with everything from minor injuries to life-threatening conditions requiring immediate treatment. Delays of four hours or more for treatment are not uncommon and in the worst performing departments most patients wait well over two hours before they are discharged, according to another Audit Commission study.[24]

The Patient's Charter requires that people 'should be seen immediately and their need for treatment assessed by a doctor or a nurse'. To meet this requirement, patients arriving in A&E are now customarily inspected by a triage nurse who assesses the nature and urgency of the case. The percentage of those assessed within five minutes of arrival rose from 75 per cent in June 1993 to 94 per cent in March 1996.[25]

But 48 of the more than 260 departments in England failed to assess 90 per cent of their patients within five minutes of arrival, according to the 1997 hospital league tables produced by the Department of Health. Eleven failed to deal with 80 per cent of arrivals in that time and two less than two-thirds.[26]

However, promptness of initial assessment does not necessarily lead to prompt treatment. In three of the A&E departments studied by the Audit Commission, almost all new
arrivals were screened within the five-minute target and seen
by a doctor or nurse who could treat them within an hour.
But others which hit the Patient's Charter target for screening were among the worst performers in actually treating patients; at one hospital less than a third were seen within an
hour.[27]

The triage system has been memorably characterised by
Frank Dobson, Labour's Health Secretary, as the appointment of a 'Hello' nurse simply to greet people arriving in
A&E. It was a sham, he said, and a cause of the abuse and as-
saults to which casualty staff were exposed.[28]

Clearly short waits cannot be guaranteed in all circumstances and most patients will accept delays when real emergencies divert staff to urgent cases. But the reasons for the
delays reveal the failure of hospitals to organise themselves to
serve their patients.

For example, many trusts appear to do little to match the
number of doctors and nurses to the average workload in
A&E.[29] Some hospitals have fewer A&E doctors on duty at
weekends *even though the number of patients is usually as great as
on weekdays*. Others schedule clinics and training sessions at
busy times of the day, causing delays to build up. Another factor identified as responsible for poor service was antique
records systems. A third of the departments studied still used
manual registration systems; of those that were computerised, some could not exchange data with other systems in
the same hospital.[30]

Perhaps the most high-profile problem of A&E depart-ments, however, is delay in admission for the 15 per cent who need treatment as an in-patient. In the worst cases, patients are left on trolleys waiting for a bed to become free or trans-ferred around the country to a hospital with a spare bed. The Patient's Charter was expanded in 1995 to include a target of a maximum delay of two hours between the decision to admit a patient and their arrival on a ward. But as the Audit Commission points out, this is open to manipulation: the de-cision to admit can be delayed until a bed is in sight; the pa-tient may be in no position to monitor progress; and the condition can be met with a series of unsatisfactory tempo-rary beds on inappropriate wards which does more damage to the patient's health than a longer wait in A&E.[31]

The Audit Commission found no simple solution to the problem of 'trolley waits' because there are many contribu-tory factors. For example, specialist doctors do not prioritise admitting emergency cases over other less pressing commit-ments, and many hospitals are too slow to deal with bed shortages as they arise.

The overwhelming message from the Commission's analysis is that hospitals have simply not geared themselves up to admit emergency patients in an acceptable manner – one of the most basic steps in the treatment of patients.

The beleaguered general practitioner
The family doctor service is, as already noted, much valued by the general public. And throughout the world, there has been a shift towards strengthening the role of what analysts call primary care in health services. This involves changing

the emphasis from secondary care in institutions such as hospitals to the general practitioner (or the equivalent in other countries).

In the UK, the strongest move in this direction has been the introduction of GP fundholding, part of the 1991 NHS reforms. As we shall see in Chapter 3, this gave selected GP practices responsibility for buying non-urgent treatment on behalf of their patients. And while fundholding is now to be phased out by the new Labour government,[32] GPs are to retain a role in buying treatment for their patients through 'locality purchasing', whereby groups of practices in an area make the decisions.

This strengthening of the GP's role reflects the importance of the family doctor service in the NHS. The general practitioner is the first port of call in the UK health service (unlike in some other countries), and GPs are responsible for 90 per cent of all health care contacts in the NHS. They also play an essential role as 'gatekeepers', controlling demand for expensive hospital facilities by screening patients.

Some general practitioners have grasped the opportunities offered by fundholding and other experiments to make big improvements in the service given to their patients. Many have used fundholding to negotiate better terms with hospitals, shorten waiting lists and provide traditional hospital services such as physiotherapy at their surgeries for the convenience of patients. The very best have turned their practices into health centres equivalent to the old cottage hospital, offering day surgery as well as a wide variety of health care services.

GPs are becoming much more professional in the way they

provide services to patients, with an enormous increase in the number of support staff employed in the family doctor service. For example, between 1989 and 1995 the number of practice nurses doubled to more than 10,000.[33] Almost all practices are computerised and some 70 per cent of prescriptions are printed on computer-generated forms.[34] Proper out-of-hours deputising services are now widely used to give 24-hours a day, seven-days a week service.

But according to the chief executive of one district health authority, the reality of general practice still falls far short of its potential:

> Too many general practices still do not offer the range of services that befits late 20th century primary health care: good health promotion, skilful counselling, expert diagnosis and apposite referral to other services where necessary, timely appointments, effective use of other primary care staff including practice nurses and nurse practitioners, chronic disease management, effective and appropriate prescribing of drugs, high-quality out-of-hours services preferably not provided by deputising services, palliative and terminal care, efficient follow-up and information to patients.[35]

One symptom of this is the number of GPs working alone or in pairs – particularly in inner-city areas. Table 1.7 shows that while there has been growth in the number of larger practices since 1985, a tenth of practices still have only one partner and just over a fifth have two.

Table 1.7
Structure of GP practices in England

No. of principals	1985	1995
1	2,915	2,794
2	3,880	3,612
3	4,986	4,041
4	4,352	4,784
5	3,610	4,345
6 or more	4,292	7,126

Source: Department of Health, *Health and Personal Social Service Statistics*, quoted in Harrison and New, *Healthcare UK 1996/97*, 1997, p. 8.

This affects only a minority of people, since the vast majority of the population is registered with family doctors working in practices of three or more partners. But single- and dual-partner practices are often concentrated in the least affluent areas – especially inner-city areas where health inequalities are most evident.

A fifth of London's GP practices, for example, are single-handed, compared with 9 per cent in the rest of England. A quarter of the premises in the capital are below the minimum standard – the figure is 2 per cent for the rest of England – and 14 per cent have no practice nurse, compared with 4 per cent elsewhere.[36]

One impediment to raising the standard of the family doctor service is the self-employed status of most general practitioners. This is a hangover from the pre-NHS days, and is strongly supported by those doctors who fear a salaried service would lack the independence necessary to do the best for patients. But it means changes in the service have to be negotiated, and are often slow to be implemented.

A small but not insignificant reflection of this independence is revealed in a 1997 efficiency scrutiny by the NHS Executive into prescription fraud, which it estimated cost up to £100 million a year.[37] The average GP prescribes drugs and other items worth £127,000 a year, but the team found few controls in prescribing practices to limit the risks of fraud.[38] While there were a few cases of fraud by GPs, most of the losses in this part of the NHS come from sloppy work practices such as:

- allowing locums and other staff uncontrolled access to prescription forms
- abuse of the repeat prescription system to issue extra prescriptions
- bad handwriting which allows prescriptions to be altered or the items to go to someone not intended to receive them.

The general practitioner is a well-respected professional who is in many respects in the front-line of the National Health Service. Considering how little of the NHS budget is consumed by the general medical service – 9 per cent in 1995 – it is remarkably good value for money. But again the question must be asked about whether it is an adequate level of service.

The best GPs are offering world-class primary care in innovative ways, reshaping the health service to meet their patients' needs. But too many are still operating in conditions that owe little to the last decade of the 20th century. And one common practice again reveals the gulf between the NHS family doctor service and the best in private sector services: the delay in seeing a GP other than in emergencies.

The introduction of timed appointments 20 or more years ago was at least an improvement on the standard practice of queuing in the doctor's waiting room throughout surgery hours. But delays of two or three days for an appointment are not unusual – and a sharp contrast to the service available from household appliance repairers or drain cleaners, to name but two.

Britain deserves better

On one level, it might be said the sorts of criticisms outlined above are just carping. The NHS provides a pretty good service at a very reasonable cost by international standards. Some people have to wait a long time for non-urgent operations, but the upside is a health service where no-one is scared off by cost and the most advanced surgical techniques are available to all free of charge.[39]

That was certainly the view of Virginia Bottomley when she was Health Secretary. In 1994, she said the NHS was remarkably cost-effective and provided good value for money. She said the 'low administrative costs of a national system financed mainly out of general taxation' served the economy well.[40] Interestingly Frank Dobson, the Labour Health Secretary, said much the same when launching the NHS's 50th anniversary celebrations in January 1998.[41]

Yet the aim of the preceding litany is to show that the NHS falls far short in the quality of its services in comparison with what most people would expect in almost any other walk of life. Some defenders of the status quo would say there is nothing that could not be cured by an injection of funds. The preceding examples suggest it would take much more than that, necessary though higher spending might be in some circumstances.

Getting the extra resources is not a trivial question, and it is one this book will look at in some detail in later chapters. But the question that needs to be answered first is the sort of health service we want. Do we want the NHS – in the words of Rudolf Klein, the leading analyst of the NHS – to be a church or a garage?[42]

The NHS has traditionally organised itself as a church, in which the medical profession is an all-powerful priesthood. The doctor decides who gets what, because he or she knows best; the patient is the grateful recipient of treatment. The same services are provided to the whole congregation, because everyone is equal in the sight of the Almighty. And if the conditions are not tip-top, at least everyone is in the same boat. Using the NHS is an act of social communion which emphasises common citizenship – it is akin to an act of worship.

But we live in a consumer society where people expect to be treated as customers with individual needs. In many other walks of life, professionals are no longer authorities to be deferred to: they are technicians whose task is to respond to the varying demands of customers. The model is the repair garage, which succeeds if it offers choice, variety and flexibility. The user can choose between diverse services – and the result is a pluralistic, multi-tier system in which there is much less homogeneity.

Table 1.8
The competing models of health care

Church	*Garage*
Paternalism	Consumerism
Planning	Responsiveness
Need	Demand
Priorities	Choice
Trust	Contract
Universalistic	Pluralistic
Single-tier	Multi-tier
Stability	Adaptability

Source: Rudolf Klein, *The New Politics of the NHS*, 1995, p. 248.

There are, of course, good reasons why health care cannot be provided in the same way as garage services. As Chapter 7 explains, these include the complexity of the nature of health care and the consequences of making the wrong decisions. But there is evidently a demand for health services to operate more like a garage in some sense. When patients take their bodies in for repair, they want to retain more control over what happens than would be the case in a church.

Yet the NHS is still an institution very much forged in the church mould. The next two chapters examine how the NHS has come to be the way it is and the attempts of the last Conservative government to make it more like a garage. The rest of the book looks at its limited success and examines the policy options for giving the British people a health service they can be proud of – not one with serious shortcomings that are forgiven because it is running on a shoestring. That means finding ways to import the best aspects of the garage model without throwing away the undoubted strengths of the church.

2: A Child of Scarcity

The National Health Service was the child of scarcity,
conceived at a time when Britain was still recovering
from the ravages of war. It has remained a monument to
institutionalised scarcity ever since.

Rudolf Klein, Patricia Day and Sharon Redmayne, *Managing
Scarcity*.[1]

The creation of the National Health Service in the mould of
a church was inevitable given the circumstances of its birth
50 years ago – in the aftermath of a terrible war. Shared suffering had been celebrated as a sign of common citizenship,
and people had learnt that scarce resources could be mo-
bilised effectively by giving them to public servants who rationed them out more or less equally. The NHS was modelled
on this war economy – 'an act of social communion, cele-
brating the fact that all citizens were equal in the sight of a
doctor', as Klein puts it.[2]

A prototype already existed in the Emergency Medical
Service, created by the Conservative-dominated National
Government in 1938 to provide free treatment should war be
declared. The arrangements included a national blood trans-
fusion service, nearly a thousand new operating theatres and
tens of thousands of beds in Nissen huts. At first it was only
for war casualties, but once hostilities began it was extended
to war workers, child evacuees and many other groups.[3]

Even before the Second World War, something of a national consensus had been established that Britain needed a
comprehensive health service, free to all at the point of use.

Free treatment had first been mooted by Beatrice Webb, the redoubtable Fabian, in her minority report to the 1909 Inquiry into the Poor Law. By 1926 the idea had entered the mainstream when a Royal Commission on National Health Insurance called for a medical service 'supported from the general public funds'.[4] In 1934, the Labour Party adopted plans for a comprehensive, free and salaried service drawn up by the Socialist Medical Association.[5]

So it is hardly surprising that a Conservative Health Minister in the wartime coalition drew up the first blueprint for a post-war health service. A white paper produced in February 1944 established two fundamental principles:[6]

- the new service would be comprehensive – 'every man and woman and child can rely on getting all the advice and treatment and care which they need . . . and that what they get shall be the best medical and other facilities available'

- services would be free, so that access would not 'depend on whether they can pay for them, or any other factor irrelevant to the real need – the real need being to bring the country's full resources to bear upon reducing ill-health and promoting good health in all its citizens'.

The consensus over the need for a free and universal service reflected the shortcomings of the existing British health insurance scheme. Introduced by Chancellor of the Exchequer David Lloyd George in 1911, it had been modelled on the social insurance system created in Germany during the 1880s by Chancellor Otto von Bismarck.

The UK scheme was financed by contributions from employees, employers and the exchequer and covered only male workers earning less than £160 a year. Members had the right to consult a panel family doctor and to sick pay, with other benefits at the discretion of the friendly societies that administered the scheme. That left most working people dependent on charity for hospital treatment – and completely excluded wives and children, the unemployed and the self-employed.

It was, however, the Second World War that converted the consensus for a free and universal health service into reality. And the circumstances of total war also managed to create a system that was peculiarly devoid of considerations of cost – a feature that was to determine the history of much of the NHS's first half-century.

A revolutionary moment

Monday 5 July 1948, launch day for the new National Health Service, has been described as one of the great days of British history.[7] Not only did it establish a health care system that guaranteed every citizen the right to the full range of medical treatment, free at the point of use: it was also the first day of Britain's new welfare state, with a social security system covering everyone from cradle to grave. It was the day when a shadow was lifted from millions of homes, according to Aneurin Bevan, the post-war Labour Health Minister who was the architect of the NHS. No longer would families have to worry about the cost of a doctor's consultation or scrimp and save to pay the fees for hospital operations.

The day was celebrated in appropriate British style. There was a political spat over Bevan's speech in Manchester the night before when he had described the Conservatives as 'lower than vermin' for opposing the legislation which created the NHS. In Edlington, South Yorkshire, a colliery band marched to the doctor's surgery and began to play, the doctor hung a Union Jack out of the window and gave them all a drink.[8] And across the country, doctors, dentists and opticians began an onslaught on the accumulated backlog of untreated conditions that was to bust spectacularly the first year's budget for the new service.

'I shudder to think of the ceaseless cascade of medicine which is pouring down British throats at the present time,' said Bevan 18 months later when faced with rapidly mounting costs.[9] But the arrival of the bills was still some way off, and Britain could instead enjoy the first dividend of post-war reconstruction.

The investment which produced that dividend had begun seven years earlier, as part of extensive preparations for reconstruction. Such planning was seen as essential in convincing those whose efforts were needed to win a total war that their sacrifices would be worthwhile – in contrast to the experience after the First World War.

With the benefit of hindsight, it can now be seen that the most important step was taken in June 1941, before either the Soviet Union or the United States had entered the war. In response to a Trades Union Congress request, the cabinet decided to set up a Whitehall interdepartmental committee to investigate the messy patchwork of sickness and disability schemes. They turned to Sir William Beveridge, an academic who had been a civil servant before the First World War when he had helped in the introduction of labour exchanges and the first unemployment insurance scheme. He accepted the chairmanship of the committee on social insurance with tears in his eyes, having hoped for a much more high-profile role in the war effort as manpower supremo.[10] But when his report – drearily titled *Social Insurance and Allied Services* – was published on 1 December 1942 it assured him a place in history that his preferred job could never have secured.

Beveridge went far beyond his remit of studying social insurance, declaring it was 'a revolutionary moment in the world's history . . . a time for revolutions, not patching'. He carried out his brief by drawing up proposals for a new National Insurance scheme paying equal benefits to all the retired, sick and unemployed, based on flat-rate contributions. But he added three further recommendations as essential building blocks for the post-war welfare state:

- a national health service available to all
- child allowances for all children
- government commitment to a full employment policy.

The Beveridge report captured the public imagination with its attack on the 'Five Giants' of Want, Disease, Ignorance, Squalor and Idleness. It was a best-seller which turned its author into a national hero – a Gallup survey in 1943 showed 19 out of 20 people knew about his plan.[11] This rapturous reception was as much a function of Beveridge's assiduous preparations for its publication as anything else. In a series of articles and broadcasts he encouraged expectations of radical change – a practice that might today be described as 'spin-doctoring'.

The coalition's response was to adopt his report in principle, leaving implementation for the first post-war government. But popular sentiment, stirred by Beveridge's vigorous promotion of his plan, wanted more. In February 1943, a parliamentary debate over the government's attitude to the report led to one of the largest backbench rebellions of the war. This was followed by a series of by-election setbacks for the Conservatives. It was clear that what the historian Peter Hennessy calls booting Beveridge 'into post-war touch' could not be maintained.

In a broadcast on 21 March 1943 entitled 'After the War', Winston Churchill effectively signed up the government to the main pillars of Beveridge. It remained the coalition's policy that the details should be put before the electorate in the election that would follow the end of the war. Meanwhile, white papers were produced on aspects of the Beveridge report such as social security, full employment and a National Health Service. Family allowances were introduced in June 1945 – almost the last act of the coalition government before the general election.

When that election resulted in a Labour landslide, there could be little doubt that the Beveridge blueprint would be implemented. Within weeks, Bevan had presented his plans to the cabinet for a free and comprehensive health service providing medical treatment to all citizens. Less than three years later, the voluntary and municipal hospitals had been nationalised, consultants had become salaried employees and a family doctor service established.

All of this was to be funded largely from taxation, with a residual insurance element in the form of a small part of the national insurance contributions deducted from wages. But there had been scant investigation of what the cost would be – as quickly became clear.

Money no object

Cost had rarely troubled the Beveridge Committee in its 44 meetings. The issue of resources to fund its plans came up in only three meetings and eight of the 248 memoranda.[12] The report concluded that the annual cost of a free health service would be £130 million – less than half the actual first-year cost.

Beveridge had faced opposition from Sir Kingsley Wood, the Conservative chancellor, who thought his report's recommendations unaffordable.[13] But such worries were brushed aside – another reflection of the wartime conditions under which the NHS was conceived and nurtured. In fighting and winning the war, conventional financial prudence had simply been put to one side. 'We threw good housekeeping to the winds,' said Lord Keynes, the economist who served as Principal Treasury Economic Adviser during the war, 'but we saved ourselves and helped save the world.'[14]

The UK had been able to achieve a 'greater degree of mobilisation of resources, human and material, than any other belligerent', as the military historian Correlli Barnett puts it.[15] The task of creating a National Health Service looked small beer for a country which had managed such a prodigious output of tanks, guns, aircraft and ships. Britain's genius for invention – exemplified in the Spitfire, radar and jet aircraft – had created a 'can-do' culture.

The myopia over costs was widely shared – as can be seen from a survey carried out during the blitz by Mass Observation, the pioneering opinion-polling organisation. It asked people about their expectations from post-war reconstruction. While 29 per cent mentioned less class distinctions, 19 per cent education reforms and 14 per cent increased social services, just 6 per cent foresaw the higher taxation that would be needed to make such aspirations a reality.[16]

In such an atmosphere, attempts to shelve the Beveridge report on the grounds of cost – or any other grounds – were doomed. But the failure to carry out rigorous financial planning for the new NHS persisted into the post-war era. In drawing up the plans for the NHS, for example, no research was done to calculate the likely level of demand once medical treatment, dental services and eye tests were free at the point of use.

PEP, the respected think-tank, had put the annual bill for health services at £161 million in 1937 – much less than a free service was likely to cost. A report in the same year by Medical Planning Research, a group of young doctors, reckoned the bill for a comprehensive service would come to £230 million a year.[17] But Bevan's first draft plan, submitted to the cabinet in December 1945, guesstimated the annual cost for England and Wales at just £145 million in the early years, with another £17 million for Scotland.

In the run-up to the launch day, estimates were laid before Parliament in February 1948 for gross costs of £198 million for the first nine months of the NHS (including Scotland). By the end of the year, it was clear there would be an overrun and the total came to £276 million – taking the bill for a full year to more than double the guesstimates produced by Beveridge and Bevan. The Health Minister then warned his colleagues that the cost for 1949–50, the second year of the NHS, would be £330 million – mostly running costs, and with very little capital investment. 'The rush for spectacles, as for dental treatment, has exceeded all expectations,' he told the cabinet:

> Part of what has happened has been a natural first flush of the new scheme, with the feeling that everything is free now and it does not matter what is charged up to the Exchequer ... there is also, without doubt, a sheer increase due to people getting things they need but could not afford before, and this the scheme intended.[18]

When the Treasury demanded £100 million of cuts (including £12.5 million for Scotland), Bevan offered a reduction of £27.75 million, mostly in capital expenditure. Less than seven weeks after the start of the new financial year, however, Bevan and the Scottish Secretary were asking the cabinet for a supplementary estimate of £57 million. The total for 1949–50 eventually came to £449 million gross, rising to £465 million in 1950–51 and £471 million in 1951–52.[19]

Thus within months of its launch, the new NHS was in financial crisis – a condition that has dogged it for most of the 50 years since. One solution was to introduce charges. Bevan conceded the principle of prescription charges in the aftermath of the September 1949 devaluation of sterling, but staved off their introduction. He also successfully resisted attempts to legislate on charges for spectacles and dentures.

But Hugh Gaitskell, the new Chancellor who was determined to get a grip on NHS spending, revived the proposals in the run-up to the 1951 budget. His success in forcing the introduction of charges for teeth and spectacles led to

Bevan's resignation and divided the Labour Party for the next decade. Charging was extended in 1952 when the new Conservative government took advantage of Labour's legislation to introduce a charge of one shilling (5p) for prescriptions and add a flat-rate charge for dental treatment. As Nicholas Timmins notes, 'within three years of its birth, the completely comprehensive and free health service had ceased to be'.[20]

In practice, however, charging was not to play a significant role in the NHS – never providing much more than 5 per cent of its income. Most of the pressure on a health service free at the point of use was to be contained by rationing – using a variety of techniques to match limited funds to much greater demand.

An age of austerity

Already on day one of the NHS, queues had begun to form. There was a shortage of dentists and a five-month wait for spectacles.[21] But in the early years, rationing manifested itself largely in austerity, in providing services that were basic – inadequate by later standards.

People accepted those conditions, however – glad to have any health service where before there had been none or restricted access. And the experience of wartime rationing had bred an acceptance across society of the shared suffering and privation imposed by total war. Britain had grown accustomed in wartime to the idea of 'fair shares' in allocating basic staples of life that were in scarce supply. The keys to the success of wartime rationing were simplicity and fairness: 'People are willing,' a report in March 1942 concluded, 'to bear any sacrifice if a 100 per cent effort can be reached and the burden fairly borne by all.'[22]

In the post-war years, Britain found itself almost bankrupt and acutely short of everything from food and raw materials to power and manufactured goods. Fair shares meant the continuation of rationing and allocation by the centre, as shops remained empty and queues pervasive. The weekly food ration in 1948, the founding year of the NHS, was as follows: less than a pound of meat, 1½ ounces of cheese, 6 ounces of butter and margarine, 1 ounce of cooking fat, half a pound of sugar, 2 pints of milk and 1 egg. (For readers under 40, one ounce is about 30g; half a pound is 225g.)

'Rationing was thought of as a *necessary* restriction during the war, and people happily turned the queue into a national institution,' wrote one observer.[23] George Mikes, the Hungarian humorist, declared queuing to be Britain's 'national passion':

At weekends, an Englishman queues at the bus-stop, travels out to Richmond, queues up for a boat [on the Thames], then queues up for tea, then queues up for ice-cream, then joins a few more odd queues for the sake of the fun of it, then queues up at the bus-stop, and has the time of his life.[24]

While there were always those who jumped the queues or found their own sources of black-market supplies, queuing was also seen as a positive element which bound people together across classes. As Ted Young, a trainee manager at the Skegness holiday camp created by Billy Butlin in the 1930s, recalled: 'it was nothing weird to see a barrister, doctors and many professional men queuing up with the road-sweeper or the refuse person, all getting together and having a very good time.'[25]

The philosophy of fair shares – if necessary, requiring restraint from those who might be able to afford to buy themselves something a little better – was to infuse the new National Health Service. Beveridge constantly emphasised in his broadcasts the need for 'equality of sacrifice', and it was clear that the post-war welfare state was about much more than simply social insurance. It was, as Peter Hennessy, a historian of the period, puts it, an equality that was 'a bonding of a common citizenship'.[26]

If there was consensus that there should be fair shares for all, there was also widespread agreement that the pressure on medical resources would not last forever. The war had shown that serious problems could be overcome by the division of intellectual labour combined with scientific research.[27] Extending the benefits of medical science to all the people of Britain would undoubtedly resolve the problems of illness and disease.

Bevan – like many contemporaries – believed the cost of the health service would diminish over the years once the backlog of need was met. Nothing could have been further from the truth.

The shifting sands

Ten years later when the House of Commons held a debate to celebrate the NHS's first decade, the limits of wartime mobilisation against disease and illness were becoming clearer.[28]

Opinion polls showed that more than 90 per cent were satisfied with the service, and most doctors were also positive about it. Bevan claimed the service was 'regarded all over the world as the most civilised achievement of modern government'. Derek Walker-Smith, the Conservative Health Minister, reeled off a list of the NHS's achievements and concluded by underlining its aim of 'the prevention and, where possible, the elimination of illness'.

But one passage in Walker-Smith's panegyric indicated a growing realisation that the NHS would not wither away as the giant Disease was slain. 'If one is less likely to die of diphtheria as a child or from pneumonia as an adult,' the minister said, 'one has a greater chance of succumbing later to coronary disease or cancer.' By increasing life expectancy, the NHS now faced increasing numbers of the malignant and degenerative diseases that many had previously avoided by premature death.

Walker-Smith's successor, Enoch Powell, identified the medical factors behind rising NHS bills as follows:

> There is virtually no limit to the amount of medical care
> an individual is capable of absorbing . . . the range of
> treatable conditions [is] huge and rapidly growing . . .
> there is a multiplier effect of successful medical
> treatment. Improvement in expectation of survival results
> in lives that demand further medical care.[29]

After the explosive growth of the health care budget in the first three years, the NHS had been held on a tight financial rein for most of the 1950s. The decade was a period of booming economic growth in which spending on public services such as education soared. But the health service grew only 3 per cent in real terms between 1950 and 1958.[30] The NHS's founders had expected the queues for treatment to shrink as the accumulated backlog of untreated illness was cleared. But the waiting list for admission to hospital remained close to half a million throughout the 1950s and into the 1960s.[31]

And in a pattern that became familiar throughout the public services, funding shortages were often bridged by cutting investment programmes. We have already seen that Bevan's first offering to the Treasury when required to make cuts in the NHS's second year was mainly on the capital side. By 1952–53, hospital capital expenditure was less than a third of the pre-war level in 1938–39. Seven new hospitals had been started in the 1930s – including ones in depressed areas such as Glamorgan and Gateshead – but it was not until the 1960s that the NHS built a hospital.[32]

A consequence of this financial stringency was that little was done about addressing the inequalities in provision across the country, which remained largely undisturbed in the first decade.[33] The Sheffield area had 9.4 hospital beds per 1,000 population in 1950, while the area covered by the South-West Metropolitan Regional Health Board had 15.1. By 1960, Sheffield had 9.1, while South-West Metropolitan had 14.2. The budgets inherited from pre-NHS days were simply raised in line with each other. In an era when extra funds were scarce, tackling these inequalities would have meant removing resources from well-provided areas – many of them Conservative heartlands in the south-east.

Some progress was made in raising the number of general practitioners in poorly-endowed areas, by stopping new practitioners setting up in well-provided ones. The proportion of people living in areas with too few doctors declined from just over 50 per cent in 1952 to less than 20 per cent in 1958. And the number of consultants was raised from 5,316 in 1949 to 7,031 in 1959, with particular growth in 'Cinderella' specialities such as psychiatry. But the numbers still fell short of the targets set in 1948.

Banging the begging bowl

Bevan had quickly identified those who worked in the National Health Service as a contributing factor to the rising costs. In 1950, he warned the cabinet that doctors had too strong a grip over hospital management committees 'and were pursuing a perfectionist policy without regard to the financial limits which had necessarily to be imposed on this Service as on other public services'.[34] It was to be a familiar refrain over the years as successive Health Ministers found themselves facing ever-increasing demands for funds from those who worked in the NHS.

The nationalisation of the hospitals had freed hospital administrators from the discipline of balancing spending against funds they had to raise from benefactors, charges or local authorities. The ministry in London doled out the money, and the way to get more was to indulge in 'grantsmanship' – a practice identified by Howard Davies in the early 1990s when he was Controller of the Audit Commission.

Davies coined the term in connection with local government, where a series of reforms in the 1980s left councils responsible for raising less than a quarter of the money they spent. The consequence was that effort spent on winning extra grants was usually far more rewarding than improving the collection of local taxes or making services efficient. And the best way to get more grants was to shout as loudly as possible about 'underfunding', backed by claims of imminent collapse in essential services.

Much the same had already happened in the health service. We have already seen in Chapter 1 how much money hospitals could save if they paid more attention to the procurement of supplies. A good example of the neglect in fund-raising is the fact that around half of hospital trusts do not bother to collect fees from insurance companies for treating victims of traffic accidents. Health department officials estimate that up to £150 million a year could be collected under the existing scheme,[35] but only around £20 million is actually collected each year.[36]

As for the health professions, they learned fast that the squeakiest wheel gets oiled first. As Rudolf Klein puts it, doctors, nurses and other providers are encouraged to 'denigrate the service . . . and to advertise their own claims for extra resources by drawing attention to the NHS's shortcomings'.[37]

Competition for resources becomes ever-sharper as specialisation increases and medicine fragments into a myriad of departments and disciplines. One indicator of this fragmentation is that more than 100 specialties are listed in a recent brochure put out by one hospital. The Royal College of Nursing lists more than 70 different specialised nursing groups.[38] They too must battle for a larger slice of the cake by proclaiming the shortages they face.

Finally, the creation of a national service did much to raise expectations about pay among health workers and professionals. At first, the NHS was quite successful in holding down pay – general practitioners, for example, saw a 20 per cent decline in their real incomes between 1950 and 1959, a period when real incomes rose on average 20 per cent.[39] But this position could not be held indefinitely and there were demands from GPs and junior hospital doctors for rises. When these were won, consultants followed suit, seeking to preserve differentials.

Other groups such as nurses and ancillary workers also became more assertive, encouraged by greater unionisation. After the foundation of the NHS, the proportion of its unionised workforce rose steadily from 40 per cent in 1948 to 60 per cent in 1974.[40] The mere fact of union membership raised pay levels during this period, particularly with the growing willingness of NHS staff to threaten industrial action.

Thus, as in many public services, ministers found themselves facing noisy demands for more resources, both to improve medical services and also to raise pay and conditions for those working in the health service. The second and third decades of the NHS saw those extra resources coming in, with the health budget rising from 3.3 per cent of gross domestic product in 1958 to 4.6 per cent in 1978.[41] But none of this had much impact on waiting lists which remained at around 600,000. Whenever they began to diminish, GPs simply referred more people on to the queue.[42]

Permanent revolution

Labour governments struggled to find extra resources to meet the demand, usually unsuccessfully. The best that can be said of the 1964–70 and 1974–79 governments was that they largely protected health budgets from public spending cuts after the 1968 devaluation and the 1976 IMF loan. Successive Conservative governments took a rather more muscular approach, with a series of restructurings designed to get a grip on this behemoth and make it more efficient.

The first attempt was Sir Keith Joseph's 1974 reorganisation to create a single administrative structure capable of planning health services and implementing change. Carried through by the 1974–79 Labour government, this turned out to be less than perfect. Apart from leaving GPs outside the new set-up, it created a cumbersome structure. There were up to four tiers in larger areas, and the emphasis on consultation and consensus made for slow decision-making.

When Margaret Thatcher came to power in 1979, her new government arrived pledging a second round of restructuring – this time to decentralise the NHS. In 1982, one tier of administration, the 90 area health authorities, was abolished and power passed down to 200 district health authorities.

Scarcely was the ink dry on the 1982 upheaval, however, when a third was on the way. Mrs Thatcher had become increasingly restive about the capacity of the NHS to absorb real increases in resources and then come back to ask for more if catastrophe was to be averted. The health service appeared impervious to the sort of curbs imposed in other parts of the public services where staff had been cut and efficiency targets used to hold or reduce spending.

She decided to expose the inner managerial workings of the NHS 'to the scrutiny of a group of businessmen who would not be easily fobbed off with bureaucratic or wimpish social welfare excuses'.[43] In early 1983 she asked Sir Roy Griffiths, managing director of Sainsbury's, the supermarket chain, to lead a four-man team to investigate. Its report, one of the shortest official reports in the history of the NHS, concluded that the health service was out of control.

'If Florence Nightingale were carrying her lamp through the corridors of the NHS today, she would almost certainly be searching for the people in charge,' was Sir Roy's memorable verdict. No one was responsible for planning or performance: 'The NHS is structured as to resemble a "mobile": designed to move with any breath of air, but which in fact never changes its position and gives no clear indication of direction.'[44]

The team concluded that the NHS needed professional managers who would be responsible for making things happen. This recommendation was, naturally, controversial among health professionals. Nurses saw it as an attack on their position in the existing management structure. Doctors viewed the arrival of professional managers as a threat to their clinical freedom, importing the alien values of the commercial world into a service where the only priority was the good of the patient.

With a majority of 146, Mrs Thatcher was not to be deflected in implementing the Griffiths recommendations. Most of the first wave of general managers came from the health service: about a quarter were doctors or nurses, and 61 per cent former administrators or finance people.[45] But 12 per cent came from outside the NHS – to the horror of those who saw them as the vanguard for the commercialisation of the health service.

The funding question

The one issue that none of these structural reforms tackled was finance. Several Conservatives had, over the years, toyed with ways of switching the public funding to private insurance – including the young Geoffrey Howe in a 1961 pamphlet published by the Bow Group, a Tory ginger group. But such far-reaching reforms were not on Mrs Thatcher's first-term agenda; in fact the NHS was protected from the onslaught on public spending that dominated her early years in office.

In 1982, however, the Treasury became concerned that public expenditure was rising faster over the longer term than economic growth, threatening to take an increasing share of national income. The Central Policy Review Staff – the Cabinet Office think-tank – was asked to look at radical options to reverse what Sir Keith Joseph had described as the ratchetting up of public spending. In line with the blue skies thinking appropriate for a think-tank, the CPRS came up with a list that included ending the inflation-proofing of social security benefits and charging for higher education. However. it was the proposed option of replacing a tax-financed NHS with private insurance and increased charges that hit the headlines when the CPRS report was leaked to *The Economist*.

Ironically, the cabinet had by then already rejected the

A CHILD OF SCARCITY

paper – and the Treasury's recommendation of a further study – after what Nigel Lawson described as 'the nearest thing to a cabinet riot in the history of the Thatcher administration'.[46] But the political furore dogged the Conservatives for the rest of their period in office with the accusation that whatever they proposed was a prelude to privatisation. It also forced Mrs Thatcher to promise to preserve the comprehensive and universal health service, free at the point of use – with her pledge to the Conservative Party Conference in October 1982:'Let me make one thing absolutely clear. The National Health Service is safe with us.'

Mrs Thatcher fought the 1983 and 1987 general elections on a firm commitment to preserve and improve the health service. And successive Conservative Health Ministers were forced onto a treadmill of demonstrating that ever-more operations were being carried out and more patients treated, as evidence that the NHS was indeed safe in their hands. NHS spending continued to rise, as did the number of doctors and nurses. Indeed, the average increase between 1978–79 and 1989–90 was 3 per cent a year in real terms. Yet it could never be enough to satisfy demand – particularly in the years when spending fell below the trend growth rate.

A 1986 report from the House of Commons Social Services Select Committee calculated that the accumulated underfunding since 1980 had been £1.325 billion.[47] It could be said that 1980 was a bogus baseline and the choice of another year – or other assumptions about what was needed to avoid underfunding – could have led to very different conclusions. But comparisons with the higher proportions of national income spent on health in other countries helped reinforce the view that the UK spent too little.

The government's reply to its critics was to claim that greater efficiency was producing higher output for the budget.[48] The critics retorted that this had been achieved at the expense of quality. More important, a series of news stories just after Mrs Thatcher had won her third term with a 100-seat majority in June 1987 highlighted particular shortages which had led to the suffering and even the deaths of individual NHS patients.[49]

In July and August, for example, increasing numbers of hospitals were forced to cancel operations because of a shortage of nurses, particularly in intensive care and operating theatres. The four Thames regions covering London and the south-east – hit by a programme to redistribute NHS funds to other regions with greater needs – warned that bed closures were inevitable. In Birmingham, limits were set on the number of new kidney patients that could be taken on. And in Leeds, a local charity run by parents of children with cancer had to stump up £5,000 to keep a junior doctor in the post over the summer.

The bad news stories continued through the autumn, with more than 3,000 beds closed in England by December.[50] A shortage of intensive care nurses in Birmingham attracted particular attention as Birmingham Children's Hospital had to cancel a series of heart operations. One baby, David Barber, had his heart operation postponed five times. In early December, intensive care cots were closed in Manchester and St Thomas's in London closed a fifth of its acute beds.

In fact there was nothing new about bed closures towards the end of the financial year. It had always been the fall-back position when budgets ran out – higher levels had been recorded in 1977 and 1978, for example. Nor had the NHS been starved of funds for 1987–88, with a 4 per cent real increase in the budget in the run-up to the election. But as Nigel Lawson wrote in his memoirs, at every prime minister's question time Mrs Thatcher 'had thrown at her case after case of ward closures, interminably postponed operations and allegedly avoidable infant deaths, all of them attributed to government parsimony.'[51]

On 6 December, the presidents of the three senior Royal Colleges – surgeons, physicians and obstetricians – issued a warning that the NHS had 'almost reached breaking point'. They added: 'We call on the government now to do something to save our National Health Service, once the envy of the world.'[52]

Ministers insisted there was no crisis, and Edwina Currie, the junior Health Minister, urged those who could afford it to use the private sector. A November white paper had proposed raising extra funds through business activities and charges for eye tests and dental checks – the latter producing a rebellion among Conservative backbenchers. But on 16 December, Tony Newton, the Health Minister, announced an extra £101 million to head off bed closures, deal with AIDS and help with storm damage after the October hurricane. As MPs left the Commons, one minister remarked: 'We can't go on like this. We will have to look at the way the health service is run.'[53]

He was right: the additional funds brought little respite. Health authorities pointed out it was a one-off measure that would do nothing to remedy the accumulated underfunding. A strike by night nurses in Manchester over special duty payments began to spread. Hospital consultants in Birmingham formed groups to 'Save the NHS', while doctors around the country took out local newspaper advertisements to explain why patients could still not be treated.

Mrs Thatcher was keen to avoid a review with so much other change under way – such as the poll tax and the Great Education Reform Bill. And John Moore, the Social Services Secretary, stuck to the line under pressure in a House of Commons debate on 19 January. But six days later, Mrs Thatcher conceded a review on BBC TV's *Panorama*. To the surprise of many colleagues and civil servants, the National Health Service was launched on a new round of soul-searching in an effort to match resources to demand.

3: When Scarcity Ran Out

The NHS was born into a working class society only
slowly emerging from war, where rationing and queuing
were symbols not of inadequacy but of fairness in the
distribution of scarce resources. It celebrated its 40th
anniversary in 1988 in what had become an affluent
consumer society where only access to work was
rationed.

Rudolf Klein,[1] *The New Politics of the NHS.*

A health service designed in the 1940s now found it necessary to begin its fourth upheaval in 15 years, one that was to
be the most radical so far. For most people – inside the health
service and outside it – the issue was money. More money
would solve the problems of waiting lists, inadequate facilities and underpaid staff. But there was, in truth, something
much deeper behind this latest crisis in Britain's best-loved
institution: it had outgrown its roots.

When the National Health Service had been founded in
the 1940s, waiting lists, basic facilities and overstretched staff
were the way in which health care was brought to the
masses. Moreover, those very features of queuing and privation were part of the culture of social solidarity and shared
hardship.

But 40 years on, Britain had changed: the proportion of
manual workers had fallen from almost two-thirds to less
than a half; home ownership had risen from 27 per cent to 58
per cent. Most British people enjoyed lifestyles and posses-
sions that would have been unthinkable in the straitened cir-

cumstances of 1948. From car ownership to consumer durables, holidays to personal services, ordinary people had become accustomed to choice, variety and responsiveness to their demands. The waiting list had become an anomaly, the queue a sign of failure.

One symptom of this new consumerism was the growth of the private health sector. Although the proportion covered by private medical insurance remained a small minority, it had almost doubled over the decade, from 6.4 per cent in 1980 to 11.5 per cent by 1990.[2] Around a quarter of the managers and professionals in the top two social classes were covered, and trade unions were beginning to negotiate for it as a benefit for their members.

But support for the National Health Service as a concept was not waning. As Chapter 1 showed, opinion polls indicated a strengthening of support for the NHS during the 1980s and demands for higher spending to support it. Even those with private insurance used the NHS for much of the time: for more than half their in-patient stays and four-fifths of their out-patient attendances.

But while the NHS could be relied upon to deal with life-threatening emergencies, the private sector offered treatment to improve the quality of life – elective surgery such as hip replacements, for example. It was the garage to the NHS church, offering consumer choice over non-medical aspects such as speed of treatment and its timing.[3]

The NHS, in contrast, was still rationing out services to patients who were treated as supplicants rather than customers. This was reflected in the way batches of patients would be booked for the same appointment with a consultant, usually at the start of the clinic session. An out-patient appointment usually involved sitting in less-than-salubrious waiting rooms waiting for the medical team to arrive. The assumption was 'that not a second of the consultant's time must be wasted but that the patient's waiting time was of no account'.[4]

It was certainly the case that more resources would be needed if the NHS was to clear its waiting lists, meet every need felt by patients and provide them with an acceptable standard of service. But that had always been true: what had changed was patients' unwillingness to wait – and the willingness of those who worked in the health service to make demands on the government as paymaster. Scarcity was no longer an acceptable explanation – and finding a better one was the primary task of Mrs Thatcher's review.

Not the Royal Commission

Previous administrations of right or left would have set up a Royal Commission, with representatives from the main groups affected and a sprinkling of the great and the good. Research would have been commissioned, papers considered and a report drawn up to maximise consensus and avoid minority dissent.

That was not Mrs Thatcher's style of government. The 1989 review was carried out by a cabinet committee involving just five ministers. The prime minister was of course one member, as was John Moore, the Social Services Secretary, and Tony Newton, the Health Minister.[5] The two remaining members came from the Treasury: Chancellor Nigel Lawson and John Major, Chief Secretary.[6] They were advised by Sir Roy Griffiths of Sainsbury's and a small group of top civil servants.

The review received submissions from a wide variety of organisations. They ranged from the British Medical Association's advice to avoid change, to a privatisation plan from the Institute of Economic Affairs, the free-market think-tank. But the review team preferred to rely on a small group of advisers – most from the political right.

Just two consultative meetings were held with doctors and managers, chosen by policy advisers for their radical views. The Centre for Policy Studies, the think-tank set up by Mrs Thatcher and Sir Keith Joseph in 1974, played an important – if unofficial – role in sifting ideas. Its new director, David Willetts, a former civil servant in the Downing Street policy unit, saw the cabinet papers throughout.[7]

Each of the review team had their own pet schemes and aversions. John Moore, then Mrs Thatcher's golden boy, wanted a health tax to make people aware of the cost of the health service. He favoured offering rebates to people who opted out of the NHS for private insurance – along the lines of the scheme for those who contracted out of the state pension scheme for a personal pension.

The Treasury opposed a health tax: it has always resisted 'hypothecated' taxes earmarked for particular purposes which could weaken its grip on public spending. Chancellor Lawson turned to the traditional Treasury solution of charging much more, pointing out that charges had raised nearly double the proportion of the NHS budget in the 1950s. But Mrs Thatcher thought charges would be desperately unpopular and favoured tax concessions to encourage private insurance. This was fiercely opposed by Lawson whose aim at the Treasury was to simplify and get rid of the distortions created by tax reliefs.

Two points quickly became clear, however. The first was that opting out would be an expensive option. The young and healthy would take their NHS rebates and go private, no doubt getting lots of extra health care at present denied them under the NHS. Those who made most use of the health service – the elderly, the disabled and chronically sick – would stay with it, but would face a much poorer service after rebates had been paid to those who had opted out. Extra money would then have to be pumped into the NHS if the headlines about waiting lists and avoidable deaths were to stop, and it would be the middle-class taxpayer who would have to find it. As in the United States, opting out would in fact mean the middle classes paying twice – once for themselves and again for the publicly-funded safety net.

The second lesson was that if health care costs were going to fall on the public purse, the National Health Service was a pretty good way of holding down the bill. The UK spent a lower proportion of its national income on health care than most other industrialised countries, and on most measures was not discernibly less healthy. A centralised health care system financed largely out of taxation was better equipped to hold down spending – and doctors' salaries – than private or social insurance schemes. As Nigel Lawson says:

> We looked . . . at other countries to see whether we
> could learn from them; but it was soon clear that every
> country we looked at was having problems with its
> provision of medical care . . . all of them – France, the
> United States, Germany – had different systems; but each

of them had acute problems which none of them had solved. They were all in at least as much difficulty as we were, and it did not take long to conclude that there was surprisingly little that we could learn from any of the other systems.'[8]

More for less

If all the options for alternative sources of finance for the NHS were ruled out, the review was left with the question of whether the money currently spent on health care could be spent better. Here there appeared to be some scope to improve the efficiency of the health service, notorious for its lack of conventional financial controls. Most people working in the NHS had little idea of the cost of anything, which meant cost-effectiveness was rarely a consideration in judging between alternative courses of action.

John Moore summarised the challenge in a speech at the time of the launch of the review:

Some districts treat only 25 patients per year in each surgical bed, while others manage 53. Even when adjusted to take into account differences between the patients treated, some districts are still treating 14 per cent fewer patients than would be expected, while others are treating 27 per cent more.

Similarly there are districts with an average length of stay 13 per cent longer than expected while others manage a length of stay almost 22 per cent less than expected.

And if we turn to costs we again find large variations.

Costs within any one group of similar districts can vary by as much as 50 per cent.[9]

Worse, there were no incentives to save money, since budgets were allocated in advance. A hospital that was particularly efficient would incur extra costs by treating more patients but get no additional resources to cover them (at least not immediately). This led to the big idea of the review: that money should follow the patient. In other words, the system should encourage hospitals to treat more people by offering them extra resources immediately.

Here the review was in luck. There was already a blueprint for how to make this happen, drawn up by an American health management specialist, Professor Alain Enthoven of Stanford University in California.[10] He dubbed it the 'internal market', in which health authorities would buy and sell services from each other and from the private sector instead of providing the full range of services themselves. In other words, health authorities would become what retail store groups would call 'purchasers', buying services for their areas from the hospitals offering the best deal in terms of 'cost, quality and convenience'.

The main obstacle to this was that the health authorities also owned the 'providers' – the hospitals and other health care services. They employed surgeons and nurses and owned operating theatres and wards, making it difficult for them to buy in, say, hip replacements from a neighbouring authority or a private company. The alternative hospitals might be cheaper, but the health authority would still have to pay the wages of staff and the costs of maintaining the unused facilities. If health authorities were to become proper purchasers, they needed to be separated from the providers.

The obvious step was to privatise the hospitals – as charities or not-for-profit organisations if making them fully commercial was not acceptable. But Mrs Thatcher's hands were tied with her pledge that the NHS was safe in her hands. So the review came up with the idea of self-governing hospitals, later to be known as NHS trusts to emphasise that privatisation was not on the agenda.

This restored the independence the hospitals had enjoyed before Sir Keith Joseph's 1974 reorganisation when they were run by boards of governors.[11] Given greater freedom – under boards with strong business representation – the trusts would seek to maximise their efficiency and meet the needs of patients in just the same way as any other organisations in a competitive market.

The third element in the review's package was the idea of giving general practitioners a role in purchasing health care services for their patients. Family doctors already played an important role as 'gatekeepers' for the NHS, choosing the appropriate treatments for their patients and referring them on to consultants who could carry them out. Two health economists, Alan Maynard of York University and Nick Bosanquet at City University, had suggested in 1984 going a step further by giving GPs control of the budgets to buy hospital services. This would help in directing funds towards those hospitals and specialists which did most to meet patients' needs, as interpreted by their GPs who were closest to them.

At the time, the idea was dismissed on the grounds that GPs lacked the skills to administer such budgets. There were also obvious objections, such as what would happen if a GP had to pay for several expensive treatments and consequently ran out of money. But the arrival of Kenneth Clarke as Health Secretary in July 1988, halfway through the review, meant the idea was back on the agenda.

A former Health Minister, Clarke was worried that it would be the administrators who would buy services in the internal market. His solution was fundholding, which would give GPs who volunteered to join the scheme budgets to buy all but the most expensive operations and treatments. To encourage fundholders to shop around, they would be allowed to spend any surplus made from choosing cheaper options on improving their practices.

The Treasury did not like the idea. It was worried about whether GPs could handle large sums of money and saw fundholding as inevitably allowing public money to leak away into the private sector. It also feared that fundholders – close to voters and usually popular figures in their communities – would be a powerful lobby for more health spending. John Major, then Chief Secretary with oversight of public spending, tried to block the scheme[12], but to no avail: Mrs Thatcher saw it as a radical move in a review that was working out too tame for her liking.

The battle commences

It took less than a year for Mrs Thatcher's review to reach its conclusions, which were published in January 1989.[13] Its title, *Working for Patients,* was designed to reach over the heads of the medical profession and win support from voters – aided by one of the ritziest publicity campaigns ever mounted for the launch of a white paper. But the reaction was nonetheless explosive, sparking off the largest battle over the NHS since its foundation in 1948.

One reason was that *Working for Patients* proposed no substantial new money – nor any suggestions as to how extra resources might be provided. This was naturally a disappointment to all those in the health service who had been campaigning to 'Save the NHS'. Instead they were faced with a white paper which had reached a rather more sinister conclusion: that the health service already had lots of money and it was failing to spend it in the right way. In other words, far from government parsimony being the problem, it was medical profligacy.

Another reason for the uproar was simple political opportunism. The Labour Party knew the Conservatives were not trusted by voters on the National Health Service and was determined to exploit this. The Shadow Health Secretary was Robin Cook, one of the opposition's most incisive thinkers and fearsome campaigners. He was determined to portray the white paper as a prelude to privatising the health service – a strategy that was highly successful judging by poll evidence.

He was helped in this by an unlikely ally: the British Medical Association, which believed the reforms would lead to the break-up of the NHS. Unusually, circumstances contrived to unify two powerful groups in the BMA: the consultants and the GPs.

The consultants opposed the proposal to turn them into employees of their local trusts, rather than of the NHS regions. The idea was to make them accountable to the managers who held the budgets they were largely responsible for spending. Thus their job descriptions would be expanded to include responsibilities for 'the quality of their work, their use of resources, the extent of the service they provide for NHS patients and the time they devote to the NHS'.

Even more explosive for the consultants who jealously guarded their clinical freedom, their merit awards would now reflect management and development of the service as well as medical skills. The review proposed putting, for the first time, the hated general managers on the committees which made awards. All clinical staff would undergo medical audit, with colleagues reviewing their practices, use of resources and the outcome for patients. Meanwhile, representatives of the medical professions were to lose their places on health authorities, which would be composed of executive managers and non-executives – many from the private sector.

The GPs saw the reforms as a reduction in their clinical freedom. Instead of being free to refer patients to any hospital they chose, they would be forced to send them to those with which their local health authority had signed contracts to provide treatment. The only way their patients could get treatment not covered by such contracts would be to bid for a share of the small budget set aside for 'extra-contractual referrals'.

The GPs were, in any case, already seething over the issue of clinical freedom in connection with government plans to include in their new contract 'indicative budgets' to rein in the fast-growing NHS drugs bill. Indicative budgets were targets for each practice on the cost of drugs they prescribed –

not hard-and-fast caps on spending but recommended maximum amounts. GPs who bust their indicative budgets would not have to stop prescribing, but if they did it too often, they might face questions about their prescribing practices.

The problem of drugs bills rising faster than medical costs as a whole had affected most western countries, and a variety of measures had been adopted to cap spending. Introducing indicative budgets was one of the less intrusive approaches – other countries had forced doctors to substitute unbranded generic drugs for the more expensive branded drugs. But the British approach was seen as another Treasury attempt to introduce cash limits for general practice similar to those for hospital services. GPs' spending is almost unique in public expenditure in not being subject to cash limits.

The BMA also argued that it would stop doctors prescribing the expensive drugs they thought necessary or lead to them turning away patients likely to need such drugs. Such arguments caused much anxiety among Britain's elderly population, who feared they would be denied drugs or turned away from those practices which were trying to keep their prescriptions bill down. Their fears turned out to be groundless when the new contract was eventually imposed in April 1990, after GPs' delegates had rejected action against it.[14]

What united all wings of the medical profession was the belief that the government was leading the health service inexorably towards treatment determined by financial considerations rather than need. In one sense, this was true, in that the internal market would force people working in the NHS to consider the costs in making clinical decisions. But financial considerations had always dictated whether treatment was available, in the form of competition between consultants and hospitals for funds, beds and merit awards.

If you lived in an area which had been less successful in bidding for resources, you were less likely to receive certain forms of treatment than if you lived in an area which was better at grantsmanship. The aim of the internal market was to allocate money more rationally – ideally so that it went to those who got the best out of their funds, not those who squeaked the loudest.

The idea that the National Health Service divorced the practice of medicine from money is 'perhaps the most important founding myth of the NHS', according to one distinguished analyst.[15] In fact what it did was largely to cut the links between the practice of medicine and the income of doctors – so doctors no longer had any incentive to exclude poorer people or provide more treatment than was necessary (as in America). But as the whole history of the NHS demonstrated, money remained the great constraint on medical practice – a fact forcefully underlined by the events leading up to the review.

However, none of this perspective penetrated the furious debate around *Working for Patients*. As Rudolf Klein puts it: 'Discussion revolved around a mythologised past (an NHS in which money did not matter) and a demonised future (an NHS in which medical practice was driven by money).' The stage was set for a show-down.

The new model health service
Clarke – always a bit of a bruiser – seemed to relish a fight

with the medical profession and pressed ahead. Indeed, he stoked the fire by accusing the BMA of opposing 'any change of any kind on any subject whatsoever'. The doctors replied with a £3 million advertising campaign to ram home their message that the only problem with the health service was that it was underfunded. This included the memorable slogan: 'What do you call a man who ignores medical advice? Mr Clarke.'

BMA leaders urged the Health Secretary to pilot the reforms in one region – an approach which Alain Enthoven had recommended in his original blueprint for the internal market.[16] But Clarke was not to be deflected and decided to introduce the reforms nationwide in one big bang as the 1990 NHS and Community Care Act.

Perhaps Clarke knew something others did not: the resignation of Sir Geoffrey Howe which led to the fall of Mrs Thatcher in November 1990 also produced a cabinet reshuffle. Clarke moved on to Education, and it was William Waldegrave who had the unenviable task of bringing the reforms into effect on 1 April 1991 – a year before the last date for a general election.

The patrician Waldegrave was a former Fellow of All Souls, less of a bruiser, more of an emollient persuader than his predecessor. Aware that chaos in the health service could lose the election for the Conservatives, he took steps to ensure a soft landing for the reforms.

Thus he insisted the first year of the internal market was to be based on a steady state to avoid an upheaval. Health authorities were to 'purchase' health care for their areas largely from the hospitals and other organisations that had always supplied it. Shopping around could wait until the new or-ganisation had bedded in.

Nor was there to be a rush for trust status among hospi-tals. The 57 first-wave trusts – just over 10 per cent of the hospitals – were those best prepared to venture into this new territory. And a manageable 306 general practices in England and Wales elected to seize control of their budgets as fund-holders.

Just as important, Waldegrave had a 4.5 per cent real in-crease in the health budget for the first year of the reforms. He used £251 million of this to reduce waiting lists for hos-pital treatment, encouraging health authorities to buy in spare capacity from the private sector. And he was also able to bolster the great London teaching hospitals when they ap-peared likely to be the first casualties of the reforms.[17]

Previously, their funding had reflected the fact that they were national institutions, treating people from all over the country. With the internal market, the funds for treatment were distributed to health authorities which quickly realised they could buy treatment more cheaply locally. This was probably good news for most patients who could be treated closer to home – but it was clear that famous hospitals such as Bart's and Guy's would quickly go bankrupt. Waldegrave pumped in extra funds to keep them afloat and set up an of-ficial inquiry into London's health services – conveniently commissioned to report once the election was out of the way.

In January 1992, Duncan Nichol, the NHS Chief Exec-utive, published an upbeat review of the first six months of the internal market. He claimed an extra 250,000 patients would be treated in the first year – a 3.7 per cent increase. And he predicted 'significant inroads' into reducing delays in waiting for treatment: for the first time in the history of the NHS, no patient would have to wait more than two years for treatment.[18]

Waldegrave was equally bullish, boldly claiming success scarcely a year after the introduction of the reforms. More people were being treated than ever before and long delays were being eliminated, he said. The number waiting more than two years for treatment had dropped 14 per cent in the last three months of 1991 alone, while those waiting between one and two years had fallen by 5 per cent.[19]

He also highlighted a survey carried out for the Department of Health into the progress of the new NHS trusts. Nearly half those who had visited a trust hospital before and after it had become a trust thought the service had improved. Overall, 96 per cent were satisfied with the quality of services.[20]

Some analysts questioned whether the government's claims of improvements in numbers treated were real.[21] There were several reasons to believe the figures might have been exaggerated:

- a change in the method of recording numbers treated appeared to have added to the totals
- since money now followed patients, there were incentives to record treatment that nobody had bothered to report before
- much of the increase could be accounted for by treatment which did not involve an overnight stay in hospital – a consequence of new surgical methods rather

than the reforms
- the increases after the reforms were largely in line with trends during the years before

Other studies – some by leading Labour Party policy advisers – were more positive about the reforms. Julian Le Grand, Professor of Health Economics at the London School of Economics, summarised the results as follows in his 1993 evaluation of the internal market:

> Many hospitals are in competitive situations. Trust managers are looking for efficiency improvements. Fundholders do appear to be obtaining quality improvements for their patients, although the extent to which this is the result of the fundholding scheme per se is not clear. Medical audit is leading to changes in behaviour by clinicians.[22]

Evidence on what the reforms meant for the health of the population was hard to come by. But the percentage of the population reporting fair or poor health was largely unchanged during this period – apart from a sharp rise among professionals. And there was an increase in the number of people visiting a doctor or an out-patients' clinic for every social group over the first three years of the reforms.[23]

A recent analysis of the impact of the reforms on the 170 acute hospitals in England concludes that those which became trusts during the first three years increased their productivity more than those which did not.[24] This replicates the experience of other countries which suggests that hospitals competing in internal markets produce greater increases in productivity than those which are centrally administered.

Perhaps the most interesting case study comes from Sweden where the health service is administered and financed by the 26 county councils. Reforms similar to those in the UK were introduced in 1991, but implemented in only a minority of the counties. This allows comparisons to be made between the eight which introduced some kind of internal market and the 18 which retained centralised budgeting. All the hospitals improved their performance on admissions per bed and in-patient surgical operations per bed after 1991 – but the improvements were much greater in those operating in an internal market.[25] As one observer noted: 'Various small and anecdotal changes ... point to changed provider attitudes ... In one hospital, it is now the patients who park their cars close to the hospital, not members of staff.'[26] Stockholm's hospitals now actively market their different approaches on childbirth to expectant parents – and some have emerged as much more popular than others.

A similar experience is reported from the Netherlands which is in the middle of a health care reform programme designed to improve efficiency and consumer choice. The result has been a much greater emphasis on the quality of health care, which has become the most important way for providers to succeed in more competitive markets.[27]

It is examples such as these which have led the Organisation for Economic Co-operation and Development to conclude that 'managed competition' offers the best solution to the problems of diverse health services around the world.[28] The main elements of this managed competition are a centrally-set budget which ensures every citizen is covered, combined with competition between hospitals and doctors to ensure the money is spent as efficiently as possible. The latter are described as 'quasi-markets' by Julian Le Grand, who has studied the approach in several British public services.[29]

Changing priorities

The debate about productivity in the NHS, important though it was, masked another important achievement of the 1991 reforms. The introduction of the internal market made it easier to put the patient at the centre of the health service.

Alain Enthoven had noted in his 1985 blueprint for the reforms that the NHS paid scant attention to the patient's point of view.[30] Since it was taken for granted that patients' needs were limitless, it was seen as a waste of time to find out what they were. And if needs were infinite and resources limited, the best people to decide how the money was spent were the doctors.

There was already a strong streak of paternalism in the British public services, reflecting the Fabian thinking which had created the welfare state. This was typified by the often quoted 1937 remark of Douglas Jay, a young Labour adviser who was later to become a minister: 'In the case of nutrition and health, just as in the case of education, the gentlemen in Whitehall really do know better what is good for the people than the people know themselves.'[31]

In the NHS, the 'gentlemen in Whitehall' delegated responsibility to the medical profession for deciding how the health budget was to be divided among the infinite demands. Inevitably, the doctors organised things to meet their needs, as the practice of block-booking for out-patient appointments

85

illustrated. A particular problem was the low priority given to operations regarded as non-urgent, which meant that waiting times of two years or more were not uncommon.

This is an issue on which patients have quite different views to doctors. A MORI poll carried out in summer 1997 for the Social Market Foundation found patients considered waiting time to be by far the most important priority in deciding who should get treatment. Treatment outcome – treating those likely to live longest – was rated lowest among the five factors suggested in the poll. A similar study carried out by MORI among health professionals found the opposite: doctors saw treatment outcomes as the most critical factor when deciding who to treat.[32]

In any rational sense, the doctors are right: if resources are limited, using money on some treatments rather than others may produce better overall health. But the health service exists to meet patients' needs – and few people want to wait long even for non-urgent operations, especially when experiencing pain or discomfort. Waiting times for NHS operations are often cited as an important motive for taking out private health insurance.[33] And the British Social Attitudes survey has found waiting times – even for non-emergency operations – listed by very large majorities as needing some or a great deal of improvement.[34]

What forced the NHS to begin to pay more attention to patients' wishes, however, was an initiative from outside the health service – John Major's Citizen's Charter. This was Major's 'big idea', aimed at making unresponsive public services treat their customers with greater respect. 'People who depend on public services – patients, passengers, parents, pupils, benefit claimants – all must know where they stand and what service they have a right to expect,' Major said when he launched the idea in March 1991.

In July of that year, the idea was fleshed out in the Citizen's Charter white paper[35] which promised each public service would have to set itself performance targets and publicise them to their users. For the NHS the targets were embodied in the Patient's Charter, published in October 1991, which covered hospital and ambulance services. They included individual appointments for out-patients and guarantees that patients whose operations were cancelled would get treated within a month of the original date. But the most significant element was the promise of a maximum two-year wait for an operation (later reduced to 18 months). Shorter delays were promised for high-profile treatments such as hip replacements and hernia repairs – those where the waiting lists were longest and the pain and discomfort greatest.[36]

None of this was popular with the medical profession which warned that setting these standards would reduce the output of the NHS. The block-booking system, for example, was said to be more efficient in ensuring a steady stream of patients for the consultant. As for the targets for reducing waiting times, they would divert scarce funds to the minor operations for conditions that were not life-threatening. Far better, the critics said, for the money to be used to treat patients with the greatest clinical need.

Whatever the opinion of doctors and consultants, however, the 1991 reforms made it possible to implement the Patient's Charter standards. Under the old centralised NHS, the government could issue targets as much as it liked, but had little ability to enforce them. With the internal market, the purchasers were separated from the providers and health authorities could write them into the contracts for purchasing health care from trust hospitals and other providers. Some GP fundholders went even further by demanding shorter waiting times than those in the Patient's Charter.

As a result, the block booking of appointments became virtually extinct and consultants were much more punctual in seeing their patients. The proportion seen within 30 minutes of their appointment time rose from around half in 1991 to 80 per cent in December 1993 – reaching 91 per cent by March 1997.[37] And progress has also been made on the vexed question of waiting times in Accident and Emergency departments, as was seen in Chapter 1 – though on this matter, the targets set by the Patient's Charter are singularly undemanding.

The period after the implementation of the 1991 reforms also saw reductions in long delays for treatment. The number waiting more than two years was over 50,000 in 1991; by the end of 1994, just a handful of specialist cases had been waiting over two years and only 3,000 more than 18 months. Those waiting more than one year fell from 168,000 to just over 50,000 in the same period – close to the number waiting more than two years at the time the reforms were introduced.

Overall numbers on waiting lists changed little, hovering around the 1 million mark. But the government could boast that the average wait for treatment had fallen from around seven and a half months in 1990–91 to just over four and a half months by the end of 1994. Half of those who found their way on to waiting lists were treated within five weeks and nearly three-quarters within three months.[38]

The tide turns

While the opposition parties ridiculed such figures, there was some evidence that public opinion was turning. Dissatisfaction with the NHS had peaked in 1990, falling quite sharply in the year after the reforms were introduced.[39] In particular, a series of surveys carried out in late 1991 and early 1992 for the King's Fund, the health policy think-tank, found dissatisfaction with the NHS had fallen by a third between August 1991 and May 1992 – with the greatest fall in the autumn of 1991.[40]

Waldegrave felt sufficiently confident to trumpet the success of the NHS reforms in the run-up to the May 1992 election. For much of the preceding decade, Conservative leaders would have chosen to campaign on almost any other issue, so certain were they that they could only lose in the health debate. Whether the Tories succeeded in winning points on the NHS during the campaign is debatable: but they seemed to have partly defused this explosive issue.

Health was one of the issues on which Labour came unstuck in the 1992 campaign, with the furore over what became known as The War of Jennifer's Ear. A party election broadcast compared one child's wait of almost a year for an NHS operation for glue ear with the immediate treatment offered to another who had had the operation privately. This attempt to show the suffering of a child unable to get a necessary ear operation rebounded when the parents and doctors involved could not agree on what had happened.

The broadcast succeeded in raising health as an issue, re-

89

minding the electorate of their mistrust of the government on health issues. But opinion polls showed the use of a real child had been seen as blatant political opportunism, leaving a bad taste in voters' mouths. Overall, The War of Jennifer's Ear reduced Labour's lead as the best party on health.

4: Unfinished Business

The Labour Party's accusation that the government was bent on destroying the National Health Service was patently wide of the mark. The 1991 reforms did nothing to change the funding of the NHS, or to alter its nature as a state-controlled, tax-financed health care system. Trapped by Mrs Thatcher's pledge that the NHS was safe in her hands, the Conservatives found themselves striving to make the health service more efficient and improve the standard of patient care.

Indeed, far from destroying the health service, the Conservatives raised its share of national income to a record level – as Table 4.1 shows. In 1979, the NHS had taken 4.6 per cent of GDP, which had risen to 4.9 per cent by 1989. With the extra funds pumped in to oil the reforms, this rose to 6 per cent in 1993 where it more or less stayed for the next four years.

Table 4.1
NHS spending as proportion of GDP

Year	% of GDP at market prices
1949	3.5
1960	3.5
1970	4.0
1975	5.0
1979	4.6
1985	5.0
1989	4.9
1993	6.0
1997	6.0 (estimate)

Source: Office of Health Economics, *Compendium of Health Statistics*, 1997, Table 2.7.

Mrs Thatcher had launched her review to stop the endless demands for more money in the health service budget. Instead, the Conservatives boosted spending by more than a fifth in real terms over four years – the biggest jump since 1979. Ministers might claim that the internal market had produced a breakthrough in the performance of the NHS, enabling them to deliver more from limited public funds. But such a large boost in those funds meant they had left nothing to chance.

When the Conservatives finally bowed out in 1997 after 18 years in office, they left behind an NHS that was as universal and comprehensive as at any time in its previous 49 years. Minor exceptions apart, it remains free at the point of use. Yet as we saw in Chapter 1, the NHS still falls disappointingly short in offering a service to be proud of.

Under the internal market, health authorities are supposed to commission services to reflect the needs of the people in their areas. The trusts are there to provide most of the treatment, with performance sharpened in a more competitive and cost-conscious environment. And the GP fundholders are cast as entrepreneurs, able to use their close relationship with patients to ginger up the system. However, none of them has achieved anything like the potential for putting patients first envisaged by the architects of the 1991 reforms.

The failure of purchasing

Perhaps the most disappointing aspect of the new internal market has been the failure of the health authorities to become successful purchasers on behalf of the populations they represent. Freed of responsibility for managing hospitals and other health care services, they are supposed to decide the priorities for health spending in their areas and arrange for it to be provided efficiently. Most have done too little to change the way budgets are spent or to shop around for the best deals on behalf of the patients they are buying for.

On setting priorities, there has been little attempt to think these through systematically – as a series of studies by the Centre for the Analysis of Social Policy at the University of Bath has shown. The survey of 1993 health authority plans, for example, found 74 per cent mentioned mental health as a priority but only 8 per cent of the money allocated for priority developments went to this service. Acute services which tended to be much lower down on the priority list received 58 per cent of the money – no doubt because it was seen as the best way to reduce the high-profile waiting lists for operations. The authors concluded that: 'Spreading the money around may simply represent a strategy for satisfying the largest number of claimants at the least cost, resulting in symbolic gestures rather than effective interventions.'[1]

The latest survey of purchasing plans for 1995–96 and 1996–97 found little evidence of 'any substantial shift in the allocation of resources between services or sectors'.[2] And a 1997 study found most authorities spent very little on investigating the needs of their areas. The average cost of 58 studies carried out by London health authorities was just £13,783.[3]

One director of public health has pointed out that even when the work is done to assess needs, it is often over-ridden by the need to keep the health service on the road:

> Towards the end of the financial year, the contracting process takes over. Large sums of money are exchanged between purchasers and providers without explicit cognisance of the health strategy or programmes.[4]

In fact, such bulk contracting arrangements have been the norm since the introduction of the internal market. They were the obvious solution in the first year of the reforms when authorities were instructed to adopt a 'steady state' approach to avoid an upheaval in the run-up to the 1992 general election. This meant sticking with the pattern of services that existed before the reforms, but specifying them in contracts between purchasers and providers.

In most cases, this resulted in block contracts – broad-brush agreements to provide a full range of health care to specified standards. These contracts could be compared with full-service tenancies, where the tenant not only rents a home, but also gets it fully equipped and serviced by the landlord.

Once the internal market was in place, however, the expectation was that health authorities would break down the block contracts and start shopping around for different services. The tenant would prefer to buy his or her own washing machine, refrigerator and cooker, and not use the landlord's cleaner, cook and gardener. But in most cases this has been slow to happen, and if anything the contracting process has become more ossified since year one, with five-year contracts between purchasers and providers increasingly common.[5]

The prevalence of block contracts reflects the weakness of

the commissioning system in the internal market – made worse by the imbalance of power between purchasers and providers. In traditional markets, the customer is king and the producer is expected to be at the monarch's beck and call. Health authorities are supposed to be the kings in the NHS internal market, but there are several reasons why they are the weaker partner in negotiating with trusts.

One is that in much of the country outside the big cities, there is only one large general hospital capable of providing the full range of health services within easy reach. The same is true of ambulance services and other treatment providers. With limited scope for shopping around, the local providers effectively find themselves in a monopoly position – able to dictate terms to the buyer.

Another difficulty is that many of those charged with commissioning health services have little idea about why or how they should go about the job. When the trusts were split from the health authorities, the best managers tended to go to the trusts which offered the greatest scope for managerial improvement (and, probably, better pay packets linked to performance).

Those left at the purchasing end were often the adminis-trators. Most had only a vague idea of how to go about the job of commissioning – as was clear at the time, from the plethora of conferences and seminars on the subject. It is hardly surprising that many of them have stuck with the fa-miliar – drawing up contracts with the local district hospital to cover what was already happening.

Often, in any case, the people who know the most about particular aspects of medicine will be working for the trusts.

A report from the Health Advisory Service on mental health services covering conditions such as Huntingdon's disease and early onset dementia found that one health authority covering a large city had no mental health specialists on its staff. And an Audit Commission report on maternity services said priorities were often set by the trusts because health authorities were failing to give a clear lead.[6]

A third problem is fear of change. An administrator who toyed with radical innovation would always be aware of one large risk: failure to find a supplier. A supermarket buyer who fails to tie up an adequate supply of fresh strawberries can always buy stock on the open market. But a health care purchaser who is too aggressive with the local general hospital could find it has gone bust, with no alternative treatment available. The result would be ignominy and exposure in the local press – a consequence which suggests the wisest course for all but the bravest administrator is to accept what the local provider offers for fear of chaos.

It is, of course, a bogus fear: a hospital that goes bust can be reopened the next day under new management – though it might take more than a day to do the business. But the nature of such fears is an illustration of the weakness of the purchasing side in the NHS internal market. And those weaknesses make block contracts attractive security, with the purchaser buying the capacity of the local provider – lock, stock and barrel.

The consequence is a reduction in the gap between purchaser and provider which is at the heart of the internal market. The health authority and the local district hospital end up playing shops with each other – pretending what they have always done has become a commercial transaction.

In fact the gap was never quite as stark as a free-market ideologist might hope. Relationships in the health service are of necessity more long-term than those of the fruit and veg market where buying the cheapest apples on the day does no harm to either party in the bargain.

Family doctors have to establish working partnerships with their local surgeons and consultants in the interests of their patients. People like to know they can get treatment at the same hospital this year as last year. There would be unacceptable administrative and other costs in shifting suppliers for small changes in service or price. And in the nature of medical practice, much has to be left to trust – it would be impossible to specify every single item involved in treatment in a contract.[7]

This does not preclude competition – after all, most commercial competition is at the margin. Few large companies chop and change suppliers, and there has been a growing emphasis in business on long-term relationships as the key to competitive advantage. But the threat of losing business is still needed to persuade even successful companies to please their customers. If the purchaser effectively makes clear there is no threat to a provider on the margin, the pressure to keep costs down and raise standards is lost. The relationship between purchaser and provider then becomes one of ensuring the orderly administration of the budget. As Rudolf Klein puts it, with his customary sharpness:

> Market competition became transmuted into managed competition: a semantic change which recognised that

health authorities were more concerned to establish long-term relationships with providers than to engage in promiscuous one-night stands with whoever offered the best bargaining. Increasingly, purchasing became another name for planning.[8]

The trusts – a law unto themselves

If the health authorities have yet to make a real impact in purchasing health care, the new trusts have certainly made their presence felt. For most patients, they have been the most visible consequences of the 1991 reforms – with new corporate identities, highly paid chief executives and patient care initiatives. And those running them have found themselves in command of powerful local institutions capable of resisting unwanted change.

Certainly the trusts have much to boast about when it comes to improving the treatment of patients. Their performance in meeting targets set by the Patient's Charter has greatly improved – as shown by the annual hospital league tables. But there remain enormous variations between trusts which cannot be explained by funding or different caseloads.

In 1997, 52 of the 400-odd trusts managed to screen 100 per cent of patients arriving in their Accident and Emergency departments within the target five minutes. But 18 achieved the target in less than 80 per cent of cases. And while some hospitals managed to admit 100 per cent of patients within three months of the decision to operate, the worst performers managed barely half.

The Health Department rates performances on a range of

targets by one to five stars to give a simple measure of success. A crude league table compiled by the *Guardian* by simply averaging star ratings shows the best trust in 1997 – Wiltshire Healthcare in Trowbridge – had five stars in every category. [9] The worst was Forest Healthcare in Essex which runs Whipps Cross hospital in north-east London and which scored an average of 2¼ stars.

The differences between outer London and leafy Wiltshire might be seen to account for some of the differences between the performance of the two trusts. But the second and third best in the league tables were Stockport Healthcare and Derby City General Hospital – both in older urban areas. And the worst performers included Milton Keynes General and the prestigious Addenbrooke's in Cambridge – both of which might have more in common with Trowbridge than Stockport.

One reason for this might be that not enough has been done to give trusts the freedom to manage their resources. Astonishingly, new consultant posts are still determined by a national committee of the great and the good rather than by those closest to local needs. And a bruising battle over ending national pay agreements – now reversed with the return of a Labour government – has left trust managers relatively powerless in dealing with the cost that makes up 75 per cent of their budgets. According to Professor Alan Maynard of York University:

> The central control of both pay and volume of labour,
> particularly doctors, reflects the power of these provider
> groups and the unwillingness of politicians to disturb

antiquated and inefficient arrangements, many of which were created before the NHS.[10]

Trusts' freedom to manage their budgets creatively is, in any case, constrained by Whitehall accounting rules for the internal market. For example, they must charge short-run average costs for each speciality – there is no marginal costing allowed. This means they cannot offer rock-bottom rates to fill up spare capacity at weekends and in the evenings.

And as in much of the public sector, trusts are expected to balance their books from year to year, with no ability to carry surpluses forward. This approach creates a bias towards current expenditure with hasty spending at the end of the year to get rid of surpluses. It leaves little incentive to find long-term efficiency savings and reduces the gains to any hospital in cutting margins. Perhaps as a result, increasing numbers are failing to meet the target of a 6 per cent return on their assets – more than half fell short in 1995–96.[11]

As for investment, it remains heavily regulated, and still subject to approval from the Department of Health. New investment has been blighted for some years by the desire to kick-start the Private Finance Initiative – the attempt to get large public service projects funded and developed by the private sector. In theory, this might have made it easier to make new investments, by raising the funds outside the public borrowing straitjacket. In practice, drawing up bids to present to the Treasury has swallowed up significant sums of money and it was only in July 1997 that the first 14 projects were approved.

But there is more than Whitehall obstructionism behind

the uneven performance of the trusts. Hospitals remain organisations which lack strong incentives to encourage better use of resources. In the words of Alain Enthoven, the architect of the internal market, managers have very little 'leverage' to make services responsive to patients because of the doctrine of clinical freedom.[12]

When the NHS was formed, the consultants accepted long-term contracts of employment and subjected themselves to spending limits imposed by the Treasury. In return, they were given the job security mentioned above and clinical freedom. This has been defined by one commentator as the right of 'a fully qualified specialist physician or general practitioner . . . to diagnose, treat and refer his or her patients as he or she wishes, within the limits of self-perceived competence and available resources.'[13]

As the same commentator adds, 'this is an elastic definition which essentially represents a claim to be unmanaged.' It has, for example, allowed surgeons to perform procedures with which they have little or no experience, to make their own arrangements for clinics and appointments, and determine the weight and type of their caseload. To reinforce this freedom, national agreements give consultants lifetime tenure and formal rights to speak out – even to criticise their employer.

The 1991 reforms have done little to address this basic compact at the centre of the UK health service. The NHS rations resources and stops the medical profession from charging patients the sort of fees that are commonplace in some other countries. In return, it interferes little in how doctors and consultants spend what resources there are.

A simple indicator of the cost of this clinical freedom is the use of medical supplies, which cost the NHS £1.3 billion a year in England and Wales. The Audit Commission study described in Chapter 1 found considerable variations in the use of 'consumables' by parts of the same trust treating a similar mix of patients. For example, one ward used on average three pairs of surgical gloves for every two patients while another used one pair for the same number. With administration sets, usage varied between 2.5 per patient on average and less than one.[14] Other Audit Commission reports have found similar variations in the use of sterile supplies and X-ray departments.

The reasons for the variation are many, but include different approaches by clinical staff which 'will seldom be questioned, or even noticed'. Most trusts do not even bother to monitor usage, and if they do, make little use of the information. In one trust, the supplier of drapes for operating theatres helped the managers save 12 per cent on costs over a year by pointing out that other hospitals were not spending as much. Luckily for this trust, the supplier saw such 'total-value service' as part of its marketing strategy.

When the internal market was introduced, it was feared the cut and thrust of the commercial world would destroy the NHS and its caring ethos. The truth is rather different: it appears to have done little to shake the cosy complacency that allows such sums of money to be wasted. And as Alain Enthoven observed, the manager who attempts to introduce changes to raise efficiency is likely to be seen as a cause of problems.[15] That is borne out by the experience of the few radicals who have attempted to do things differently, and have been pushed aside by the combined firepower of those interests most threatened.

The first was John Spiers, the chairman of Brighton Healthcare NHS trust who had championed patient power. He was ousted in September 1994 after a vote of no confidence by the consultants following an interview in which he attacked doctors as meddlesome and dangerous. Few doubted the real reason was his outspoken advocacy of the rights of patients. He had, for example, tested the Royal Sussex County Hospital – and found it wanting – by taking himself into the Accident and Emergency department in a wheelchair. And he had appointed a Patients' Advocate to promote the interests of the users.

His departure was followed by some other high-profile supporters of the reforms. They included James Rawson, chairman of Burnley Healthcare Trust, following the earlier departure of top directors. Doctors, who had opposed the original application for trust status in 1991, had criticised the management style and threatened votes of no confidence in the board.

Amazingly, however, none of the managers running trusts which have gone into deficit or failed to deliver adequate service have faced equal public ignominy. Only one trust has been wound up in the six years of the internal market – Anglian Harbours NHS Trust, based at Great Yarmouth in Norfolk. It was dissolved on 31 August 1997 after it had lost contracts to its neighbours.

In these circumstances, the assets of the trust revert to the Secretary of State who can install a new manager or sell them to more successful trusts. Clearly dissolution should only be a final step, but it is not one that should be avoided: it does, after all, allow badly managed assets to be put back into use by a new management.

More important, it provides an incentive to avoid financial problems: in the NHS, trusts believe they are too important to be allowed to fail. As long as there is a drip-feed of cash to bail out those that persistently overspend, the health service will go on overspending – and still come back for more. But letting trusts limp on means those assets continue to be underused, which also means ward closures and other headline-grabbing failures.

The difficulty of making changes in hospital services has been increased – paradoxically – by the purchaser/provider split. The NHS trusts have turned out to be powerful organisations, determined to defend their empires. They are largely focused around local general hospitals which enjoy vociferous support in the local community from people who work in them, people who have been treated by them and those living near to them.

New ways of providing health services might improve things for all three groups of stakeholders. But there is no equivalent bunch of supporters willing to protest and agitate for a hypothetical future. As one purchaser said: 'There is a lot of support for the status quo and the providers always seem to be several step ahead of purchasers in rallying the support of the press and the local community to stop any changes.'[16] Or as another close observer put it:

People assume that health care is of a uniformly high standard and always will be, regardless of how it is

organised, so long as enough money is put into it.
Inadequacies are attributed to lack of money rather than
poor methods of organising and managing care ... the
general public remains generally satisfied with the care
they receive, but are fearful of erosion of a public service
and of cuts in local health care delivery. Most people
have absolutely no idea of the reasons why services
should change.[17]

A symptom of this is the opposition that invariably greets
any proposal to reduce the number of hospital beds in an
area. All the evidence suggests the number of beds needed for
acute treatment – as opposed to long-term care – is diminishing. New methods of treatment allow much more to be
done in the form of day surgery without an overnight stay.
Even when in-patient operations are needed, the length of
stay is shrinking – from an average of almost nine days in
1980 to five today.[18]

In England, the number of in-patient days in acute hospitals fell from just under 49 million in 1981 to just under 46
million in 1991 despite a 50 per cent increase in the number
of completed treatments.[19] Health economists in California
– in a country where there is no scrimping on health spending – estimate that 2.5 hospital beds per 1,000 population is
adequate. With 2.97 beds per 1,000, the NHS in England has
about 20 per cent more beds than it needs.[20]

The main obstacle to reducing the number of hospital
beds is the shortage of support for patients – especially the
elderly – who need care after discharge from hospital. In the
absence of adequate aftercare provision, such patients remain

in hospital, filling beds that could be better used to treat others. This 'bed-blocking' can be solved only by diverting resources to the care of discharged patients in the community – as the Labour government has recognised.

In fact, there is something of a Greek tragedy here: the trusts have had the misfortune to gain their independence in an era when they are in decline. Across the world, numbers of long-term hospital beds are diminishing as health care shifts from large institutions to primary care in the community. The immediate future for trusts is therefore bleak: they face a world of downsizing and restructuring familiar to many in the private sector in recent years.

But it is a future most are determined to resist. As one observer put it: 'many trust managements have been putting their energies into fighting for their existence rather than developing innovative and high-profile new services.'[21]

The disappointment of fundholding

Perhaps the biggest disappointment of the 1991 health service reforms lies with GP fundholding – the attempt to move control of Britain's health care system closer to the patients by letting family doctors buy it for them. This has produced some real benefits for patients with fundholding GPs, and those benefits have in many instances been passed on to patients not covered by the scheme. But it has failed to deliver anything like the potential in terms of creating a health service attuned to the needs of its users.

Fundholding was the most contentious of the three elements in the Conservative NHS reforms, not least because it was initially opposed by the medical profession. Critics feared it would lead to 'cream-skimming', as GPs refused to treat older and chronically sick patients in order to stay within their budgets. Many family doctors wanted neither the bureaucracy involved in holding a budget, nor the responsibility of saying no to some of their patients. They worried they would be forced to take decisions about their patients other than on clinical grounds.

However, the system was cleverly structured to meet such concerns. Fundholders were not expected to budget for the more expensive forms of treatment costing over £5,000 (subsequently raised to £6,000), nor for emergency treatment. This meant the budgets covered around 20 per cent of their patients' hospital and community health care by value – and then only the more predictable and manageable forms of treatment. The health authorities would pick up the tab for the more expensive and less predictable operations.

Second, GPs joining the scheme were given an allowance to cover management and computing costs – enough to employ someone to handle fundholding. Only the largest and best-organised practices with at least 9,000 patients were initially allowed to join the scheme. (The minimum size has since fallen to 5,000, with a cut-down version for those with as few as 3,000 patients.) And savings had to be ploughed back into the fundholders' practices, to extend or improve them – for example, by upgrading surgery premises, employing extra staff or buying equipment.

Once the scheme had been launched, it quickly became clear that most of the fears of opponents were not justified. The first fundholders used their budgets to improve services to patients – for example by paying for physiotherapy clinics to be provided in their surgeries rather than at hospitals. They also demanded higher standards from the trusts in terms of waiting times – often negotiating on a case-by-case basis rather than the block contracts adopted by many health authorities. Some even arranged for consultants to carry out day surgery in their practices, turning them into polyclinics for the greater convenience of patients. And there was no evidence of cream-skimming – the altruism of the medical profession seemed to have scored a success.

Fundholders also appeared to be effective in containing cost increases with no apparent detriment to their patients. One study of a sample of practices in the Oxford region found fundholders were better at controlling the number of patients referred to specialists.[22] There was no fall-off in the number of patients referred to specialists when GPs became fundholders – the number of referrals continued to rise as for all family doctors. But the number of referrals by fundholding GPs was increasing far more slowly than those by non-fundholders.

Several studies have shown a similar pattern in the cost of drugs prescribed by fundholders, which is rising more slowly than those of non-fundholders. This is achieved not by prescribing fewer items, but by making greater use of cheaper non-branded drugs to reduce the average cost per item. One study of more than 300 practices covering almost all the people of Northern Ireland found fundholders increased their rate of prescribing cheaper generic drugs by 13 per cent in the first year of fundholding.[23] In case this was because the fundholding practices were already better at containing costs, the study looked back to before they became fundholding –

and found the differences opened up only on becoming fundholders.

These advantages of fundholding were quickly appreciated by those who might have been most sceptical about the project. An early evaluation by Howard Glennerster, Professor of Social Policy at the London School of Economics, found fundholding had led to a 'shift in the balance of power back to general practice for the first time this century'. Although there was a danger that fundholders might leave some groups of patients high and dry, this had not happened. Individual family doctors with control over budgets were using it to force hospitals to meet the needs of their patients by delivering test results faster, providing consultations and counselling in the GPs' surgeries and being more responsive to patients.[24]

While the medical profession had opposed fundholding at the start, more than half of all practices had joined the scheme by 1997. As Merseyside doctor, David Colin-Thomé, puts it: 'The GP is the person who is in the most advantageous position to make clinical and overall judgements, and to have the power to put them into effect . . . GPs, being closer to their patients and being clinicians, seem to make much more effective purchases.'[25]

Despite these benefits, however, fundholding has remained contentious politically, and abolition formed a central part of the Labour government's December 1997 white paper.[26] The main criticism is that it has produced a two-tier health service in which patients of fundholders face shorter waiting times than those of non-fundholders. This has been seen as a direct challenge to the egalitarian principles at the heart of the NHS.

The charge of 'two-tierism' is heard most loudly towards the end of the financial year, when health authorities have run out of funds. Trusts which have completed their health authority contracts for non-urgent operations refuse to treat any more patients covered by those contracts unless further payment is made. As a consequence, the only people who can have non-urgent operations are patients of fundholders who still have some money left. The critics say that fundholding allows some patients, in effect, to queue-jump irrespective of medical need.

There are two issues of fundamental philosophical importance here. The first is that if fundholding produces a better service, the best way to avoid charges of 'two-tierism' would be to make all family doctors fundholders. That would raise everyone to the standards of the best – the argument pursued by the last Conservative government. It extended the scheme even to smaller practices so that more than half the population was registered with fundholders by the time of the 1997 general election.

The second issue is whether the benefits enjoyed by fundholders' patients have been achieved at the expense of the rest of the population. If fundholders received an unfair share of the family doctor service budget, it could be a possibility. But there is no clear evidence this has happened, according to a study of the literature on fundholding.[27]

Supporters of fundholding argue the benefits have spread to patients of non-fundholders. Where trusts have adopted new ways of working in response to fundholders, they have often extended them to all their patients. Health authorities have copied fundholder innovations for all their patients in drawing up contracts for the provision of treatment. As Nicholas Timmins, Public Policy Editor of the *Financial Times*, says:

> As with so much else that the best of fundholding has achieved – such as getting physiotherapy out of hospital and into GPs' surgeries – yesterday's advantage for a fundholder became today's advantage for non-fundholders.[28]

These gains are certainly welcome, but the disappointment is that they have been rather modest. Fundholding appears to have fallen short of its architects' aims of making the NHS more responsive to its patients. It has, for example, had little or no impact on matters of patient choice, such as which hospital they are referred to or which consultant is used.[29]

A 1996 Audit Commission report provides a critique of fundholding's underperformance that has angered many supporters of the project, but which bears rational examination. It found, for example, that only a minority of fundholders had used their budgets to organise out-patient clinics in their practices to save patients having to travel to the hospital. Most fundholders have not tried to use the freedom given to them to develop services closer to their patients.

Only a handful had negotiated lower prices, a higher rate of day surgery or direct access to operations, such as hernia or vasectomy, without the need to attend an out-patient clinic. As for waiting times, a quarter of the fundholders had not set targets for maximum waits, while half had simply adopted the targets set by the local health authority. Even in the latter case, fundholders had often failed to hold trusts to the targets.

Most fundholders had used fundholding to change the hospitals they referred their patients to – normally back to the ones they had used before the health reforms gave the decision to health authorities. But most offered their patients no choice when picking a hospital or other treatment provider. Thus it is hardly surprising that another survey found four out of five patients did not even know their GP was a fundholder. The Audit Commission concluded:

> The best-managed and outward-looking practices
> achieve most benefits for their patients . . . A few
> fundholders have made achievements across the board
> and are at the leading edge of purchasing; but the
> majority have achieved only a small proportion of the
> benefits potentially available for their patients.[30]

Fundholding has created extra bureaucracy and paper-work for hospitals and the other health organisations GPs deal with. It is clearly more complicated for trusts to work with dozens of GP fundholders than with one or two health authorities. And those fundholders who take the idea of shopping around seriously generate more work for trusts than health authorities buying treatments en bloc.

In practice, this should be seen as a criticism as much of trusts as of fundholding. Proper systems of pricing and invoicing should make it easy to cope with multiple buyers.

That is, after all, what happens in much of the rest of life where consumers customarily shop around for single cars, appliances or houses.

But even ignoring the extra costs generated for trusts, the Audit Commission found the scheme had cost more than the savings fundholders had accrued from it.[31] It found efficiency savings of £206 million by the end of 1994–95, compared with the £232 million given to fundholders for the extra costs of fundholding – management, administration and computing.

Any additional costs imposed by the scheme on trusts and health authorities are excluded from these figures. So too are the improvements in the quality of service, in terms of shorter waiting times, better facilities, treatment closer to home and so on. But it is clear that these are not as large as might be hoped, or is claimed by supporters who focus on those pioneering first-wave fundholders who used their new-found freedom to turn the local health services upside down.

One additional finding of the Audit Commission report was revealing: the earliest wave of fundholders tended to achieve much more than the later ones. This is not surprising: the most entrepreneurial and imaginative GPs will have seen the opportunity to do something new and exciting, and applied in the earlier days. But the report also indicates why later applicants have been less inclined to use the scheme to patients' advantage. The commonest reason given for becoming a fundholder – cited by more than two-thirds – was that the GP saw fundholding as 'the way things are going' and 'jumped before being pushed into it'. Better patient care came second ('to improve services at local providers' – 56 per cent) and fourth ('to shorten specific waiting times' – just under 50 per cent). But third at just over 50 per cent was to improve referral freedom, while five and six also related to the management of the practice rather than better patient care.

The truth is that only a minority of GPs who became fundholders were strongly sold on the idea of using the scheme to raise the standard of patient care – most went into it for defensive reasons. This explains why the benefits for patients have been so limited.

Where's the patient?

The NHS has thus been converted into a far-from-perfect internal market. Health authorities commission health care on apparently flimsy grounds without any clear view about their role. The trusts continue on their own sweet way, run by the medical profession for their convenience and using their local popularity to fend off change. And while some GP fundholders have made great strides on behalf of their patients, a lot more have made disappointing use of their new freedom.

The result is the UK still falls far short of providing the sort of health service its people are entitled to expect – one that is responsive to patients and efficient in using resources. The church may have been reorganised to mimic the sort of buying and selling that goes on in the garage market, but it remains at heart a church.

Ironically, critics of the 1991 NHS reforms are still likely to characterise them as having introduced the ethos of the commercial world into the medical sphere. It is hard to imagine any sphere of commercial life where the preferences of the individual user are given so little weight. The free market may be distorted by monopoly, the manipulation of consumers and shady business practices. But one thing is clear: a consumer with money to spend is treated as the centre of attention and offered the chance to make choices – however partial – in a way that is quite alien to the NHS. As Professor Alan Maynard of York University says:

> The consequence of the policymakers' incomplete comprehension of the need for a 'competition package' was that with great effort, the Thatcher government 'lurched' the NHS towards a competitive system but fell far short of achieving this goal . . . Consequently there is a risk that the reform process has created a quasi-centralised bureaucratic confusion dressed up in the rhetoric of market competition.[32]

The extent to which that confusion would lead to the next crisis in the health service was not obvious in the early years of the decade. But as the 1990s wore on, it quickly became clear that the 1991 reforms had done no more than provide a breathing space in the struggle with the central problem of the NHS: how to raise the resources for health care and allocate them in a situation where the gap is continually widening between expectations and what is available.[33]

5: Paradise Postponed –
The Coffers Empty

The boost to the NHS budget in the years immediately after the 1991 reforms ensured that the gap between resources and demand continued to close, at least in terms of waiting lists. But such increases could not continue indefinitely, especially as the government was struggling to cut public sector borrowing in the aftermath of sterling's ejection from the European exchange rate mechanism in 1992. A series of tough public spending rounds from 1995 onwards meant the pressure began to build again in the NHS during the run-up to the 1997 general election.

The Conservatives stuck to their pledge of real growth in the NHS budget every year. But the scale of the increases fell well below the 3 per cent a year average since 1979. For hospital and community health services, the real increase fell to 1.3 per cent in 1995−96 and 1.1 per cent in 1996−97 − compared with 6.9 per cent in 1991−92.[1]

This throttling back came at a time when other factors were adding to the pressure on the health service. There had been a sharp rise in emergency admissions − up by 13 per cent in four years. And the introduction of shorter working hours for junior hospital doctors had added to the salary bill.

By the time of the 1997 general election, waiting lists had begun to grow fast − reaching 1.13 million at the end of March 1997. By December of that year, they topped 1.26 million, 14.2 per cent higher than the year before. While extremely long waiting lists were still under control − only 974 patients had been waiting longer than 18 months − the number waiting over a year had risen from 22,200 in December 1996 to 67,370.[2]

Now the pressure for more spending fell on a Labour government pledged to reduce waiting lists. Labour's pledge on this was, in fact, modest. One of the ten pledges made by Tony Blair as benchmarks for the electorate to judge him on, it promised to reduce bureaucracy in the internal market in order to release funds sufficient to cut waiting lists by 100,000.

That was certainly achievable, though whether the cuts in bureaucracy – largely generated by reducing competition in the internal market – would help was a moot point. But perhaps rashly, an election poster appeared to go further by declaiming 'Waiting Lists Will Be Shorter'. Whatever Mr Blair had promised in the manifesto, expectations were rather higher.

The obvious course was to throw money at waiting lists – just as the Conservatives had done in the months after the introduction of the 1991 reforms. Labour had no such option, however. It had promised the electorate it would stick to the public spending totals set by the Conservatives. This promise – combined with the pledge not to raise tax rates – was seen by party strategists as essential in reassuring 'middle England' that New Labour had finally broken with its old tax and spend ways. But it locked the new government into some pretty tough spending targets – with those for the health service among the most stringent.

It was clear that without new money, the NHS was heading for a crisis. Many trusts had begun to build up deficits to avoid lengthening queues for non-urgent operations. By the end of the 1996–97 year, trust debts totalled £350 million[3] – more than 1 per cent of hospital spending. Some 69 of the 100 health authorities started the 1997–98 year in debt, as did

125 of the 425 trusts.

The outlook for 1998–99 was even bleaker – the Conservative government had pencilled in an increase in NHS funding of just 0.2 per cent. Undoubtedly the Conservatives would have raised the 1998–99 figure during 1997–98, using any surplus in the contingency fund to do so. But it looked difficult for Labour – hemmed in by its spending pledges – to do that. In June 1997, Frank Dobson, the new Health Secretary, warned the annual conference of health service managers that the coming winter would be harder than the previous one, with little prospect of extra money.

In fact, Labour's first budget in July 1997 did conjure up an additional £1.2 billion for the health service from the contingency fund. Health service managers were urged to take this increase into account immediately. In other words, they should allow deficits to grow a little more in 1997–98, knowing extra money would be in the pipeline for the next year.

A further £500 million was found in the March 1998 budget, raising the real increase in NHS spending for 1998–99 to 2.3 per cent. The mild winter appeared to have avoided a crisis and the return of the sort of headlines which had forced the 1987 Thatcher government to launch its review. But even with the extra money stumped up by Gordon Brown, the chances of making a substantial inroad in waiting lists looked dim without the sort of 3 per cent real annual increases those working in the NHS believed necessary.

Indeed, the view that such hefty yearly increases were needed had been quantified in the mid–1980s by Barney Heyhoe, then Conservative Health Minister. He told a Commons Select Committee that:

> One per cent is needed to keep pace with the increasing number of elderly people; medical advance takes an additional 0.5 per cent and a further 0.5 per cent is needed to make progress towards meeting the government's policy objectives (for example, to improve renal services and to develop community care).[4]

Adding a bit on for good luck had produced the rule of thumb figure that the health budget needed to rise by 3 per cent more than the rate of inflation simply to maintain standards. Yet a careful examination of each of the three engines of NHS spending – age, technology and higher quality service – shows that behind all three lies a common factor.[5] There is one simple driver for the increase in medical bills, and it is unlikely to be contained by the sort of rises voters have seemed willing to support in recent years.

Shall age wither them?

It seems almost self-evident that health spending will have to rise as people live longer. The over–65s already account for more than 45 per cent of total health spending in the UK. And the number of people aged 65 and over is expected to rise from around 9 million people to almost 15 million over the next 50 years. So the NHS budget will have to increase to fund the spending needed to care for this growing elderly population.

In fact, an even more alarming picture can be drawn by looking at the numbers of very elderly people over 85. They will more than double over the next 50 years, from 900,000 to over 2 million. And as Table 5.1 shows, health spending per capita rises sharply after 65, at 85-plus reaching seven times the amount spent on a young adult. Projecting such figures into the future produces estimates that health spending will have to rise by 3 per cent for each percentage point increase in the fraction of the population over 65.

Table 5.1
Health spending per head by age, 1993–94

Age	Hospital and community services	General practice	Total
	£	£	£
Births	1,762	218	1,980
0–4	374	157	531
5–15	185	129	314
16–44	241	147	388
45–64	356	147	503
65–74	703	249	952
75–84	1,280	353	1,633
85+	2,260	353	2,613

Source: Anthony Harrison, Jennifer Dixon, Bill New and Ken Judge, 'Can the NHS Cope in Future?', *BMJ*, vol. 314, p. 139.

The belief that health care costs will rise inexorably as the population ages is reinforced by post-war experience. Health spending has rocketed in most western countries over recent decades, at a time when the population has rapidly aged. Between 1960 and 1994, the proportion of the population over 65 in the countries that belong to the Organisation for Economic Co-operation and Development increased from 9.4 per cent to 13.5 per cent. During that period, health spending per head rose by 460 per cent compared with a 230 per cent rise in average per capita income.

But while such figures suggest that an ageing population consumes more health care, the growth in health expenditure has little to do with the increase in lifespan. A study of health spending in 20 OECD countries between 1960 and 1988 shows that the growth in health expenditure has been caused by increasing wealth.[6] As incomes have risen in the advanced economies, their peoples and governments have spent more on health services.

Once rising incomes are taken into account, there is no discernible correlation between the age structure of a population and health care spending. Countries with older populations are neither more nor less likely to have higher health spending in terms of share of GDP. Denmark, for example, has a population that is already more elderly than America's will be in 25 years' time yet spends half as much per capita.[7]

Nor has growth in spending increased where the population over 65 has grown faster. Another study of several European countries found little increase in the proportion of spending on the elderly at a time when their numbers were rising. In some countries, the proportion of the budget for those over 65 has actually fallen as their numbers have increased.[8]

The idea that ageing leads to higher health spending is simply a logical fallacy – the fallacy of composition.[9] Because individual old people incur higher health costs on average, it is assumed that health costs will be higher when the whole population ages. However, what is true for the individual is not necessarily true for the whole. As a nation ages, people change their behaviour, making different choices about how they spend their money and their health priorities. Projections based on present patterns of spending may therefore be wrong.

There are also medical reasons why the present pattern of spending among the over-65s cannot simply be projected into the future. People over 65 have higher individual medical costs because they are in the last years of their lives – when most health care is needed. One American study found that 18 per cent of the medical bills in a person's lifetime are run up in the last year of their life.[10]

If people live for 20 years after 65 rather than 10, at least some of the extra years will be healthy ones. People living until they are well into their eighties do not suffer the illnesses in their sixties and seventies that afflict people who die in those decades of their lives. As one observer puts it, older people remain reasonably healthy and independent until a final trauma takes them off – a model described as 'terminal drop'.[11]

In the nature of things, elderly people will suffer more illnesses as their lifespan increases. But these are likely to be light-to-moderate disabilities with fewer severe ones.[12] The annual General Household Survey reports no significant increase in the proportions of over-65s reporting limiting longstanding illnesses during the last 20 years (though, interestingly, proportions have risen in younger age groups).[13]

There is no automatic escalation of costs in proportion to increasing longevity.

Thus the most pessimistic calculations for the OECD countries suggest that ageing will add 0.8 per cent a year to health spending between 1990 and 2015. More optimistic assumptions about the amount of health care the elderly consume produce an annual increase of health budgets of just 0.3 per cent a year in real terms.[14]

Ageing is a seductive explanation for rising health care bills because it is something beyond human control. As the author of the study which demonstrated ageing has little impact on health costs put it: 'By making it seem as if cost increases are inevitable, attention is diverted from the real and difficult choices that must be made.'[15]

Believing that an ageing population gobbles up much more in health care suits those who argue that the solution to the problems of the NHS is to pump in more money. But they are wrong – increased wealth drives up the bills, because it leads patients to demand more from the health service.

The cost of tomorrow's world

If elderly people cannot be blamed for rising health bills, then how about the cost of expensive new forms of high-tech treatment? Medical innovation is seen by many as the greatest influence on rising health care costs, not least with the arrival of new generations of pharmaceuticals that can prolong life provided someone is prepared to pay the cost. The highest profile example is beta interferon, which appears to benefit some multiple sclerosis sufferers and costs around £10,000 a year per person treated.

A similar effect is noted with new forms of treatment which mean previously hopeless medical conditions can now be cured. For example, transplant techniques have become commonplace for kidney complaints, liver diseases and heart disease. Premature babies born more than 10 weeks early routinely survive thanks to new techniques, drugs and equipment. Tiny electronic devices can prolong life and artificial organs replace worn-out body parts such as heart valves. None of these come cheap.

Electronics has also provided a new generation of diagnostic equipment, such as the £500,000 CAT scanners which can help find tumours in patients and which every hospital wants access to. Ultrasound devices can scan babies in the womb and help eliminate gallstones without surgery. Lasers now have more and more uses in medicine, including bone surgery and clearing clogged heart muscle channels.

Since we live in a global village, knowledge about what is going on in other countries is transmitted widely and rapidly. Patients and their families know about the latest pharmaceuticals and operations and expect to have access to them. It is no longer an option for the National Health Service to rely on ignorance to hold off the arrival of expensive new treatments.

But expensive though many of the new devices and drugs are, technology does not invariably mean higher costs. There are also great savings to be made by developments in prevention and treatment. For example, some drugs control conditions more cost-effectively than much more expensive operations or therapies. The conquest of tuberculosis is a good example: a few pounds of antibiotics saves the three or four years' treatment in a sanitorium that was once standard. Hundreds of mental health institutions have been closed thanks to anti-psychotic drugs. And while the latest AIDS drugs may cost £5,000 a year or more, keeping the patient in hospital can cost that much for a week.

Vaccines have effectively eradicated illnesses such as poliomyelitis which afflicted thousands every year in the 1950s. Fluoridation of water and toothpaste has led to an enormous improvement in general dental health. And miniature equipment and fibre optics have created the new type of keyhole surgery which is much less intrusive for the patient. As a result, many of the operations which previously required several days in hospital can be done without an overnight stay. This has contributed to the fall in average length of stay in NHS hospitals from 36 days in 1960 to seven days by 1995.

Much of this reduction is due to the closure of the long-stay hospitals and a shift to care in the community. But even in the treatment of acute specialities, the average stay is around five days – half the figure 20 years ago.[16] As a result, the number of people treated in hospital has more than doubled from 4.7 million in 1960 to 9.4 million in 1995, but the number of beds per 1,000 of the population has more than halved.[17]

Further savings could come from developments in information technology and telecommunications. Three-quarters of the cost of the NHS is the wages and salaries of those who work in it, providing a labour-intensive service that has seen increasing payrolls at a time when most other industries have reduced their staff costs. The internet and video links which will allow consultations and diagnosis at home or local health centres could enormously reduce the cost of 'distribution' in health care.

As in many other services, much more processing will soon be done locally in GPs' surgeries or even at home rather than in hospitals which are the equivalent of the old, centralised, mass production plants. Desktop laboratory analysers, for example, could reduce the number of people needing to go to hospitals for tests. Diagnostic kits have already largely replaced laboratory pregnancy testing and might soon allow patients to identify or control a wide range of conditions.

Further in the future, genetics may make it possible to reduce the wear and tear on the human body at less cost than the current maintenance programme. Silicon chips which scan genes to detect illnesses are already under development, as are devices which can change them to treat or prevent the illnesses. According to John Bell, Nuffield Professor of Medicine at Oxford University: 'Genetics research will have the most significant effect on our health since the microbiology revolutions at the end of the 19th century'.[18]

Finally, while new and often costly drugs are added to the prescribers' lists every year, the cost of others falls. And the trend towards selling more pharmaceuticals over the counter in chemists' shops relieves the burden on the National Health Service. Simple advice from pharmacists able to dispense medicines can be much cheaper than consulting a doctor to get a prescription – and may be no less efficacious.

Indeed, the assumption that new technology automatically means higher costs is not borne out by experience from other walks of life. Modern information technology, for example, has allowed consumer companies to reduce the bill for processing paperwork and serving customers. The real cost of many household appliances and electronic equipment has fallen over the years. And cheaper food has followed in the wake of scientific developments in breeding, cultivation and processing.

In some cases, lower unit costs encourages higher spending overall. This can be seen in computing where the cost per megabyte of Random Access Memory has fallen, as has that of the 'megaflop', 1 million floating point operations. But advanced economies are spending ever-larger amounts on personal computers and computing services, despite lower prices for the components and software.[19]

In medicine, the arrival of cheaper forms of medical treatment often leads to an increase in the number of people treated – as can be seen in the NHS output figures. And if one type of treatment becomes easier and cheaper, doctors may just offer more of other, more expensive, courses. In dentistry, for example, the number of fillings and extractions has plummeted in recent decades, but there has been no let-up in the level of dental treatment. Dentists have simply offered alternatives such as cleaning, straightening and other more cosmetic operations.

But there is nothing inexorable about technology forcing up health costs – any more than an ageing population inevitably means higher bills. Health care spending can rise when technology advances because that is how people choose to react to changes in relative costs. And in a more affluent society where people have higher expectations from the health service, they demand more when it can be done.

But these are factors within the control of patients and health professionals. The fact that ageing and technology are both blamed for the rising cost of the NHS allows people to avoid the more complex issues that arise as societies become wealthier and the medical profession is able to offer an ever wider range of treatments.

Improvements in services

The third factor cited by Barney Heyhoe in 1986 for rising NHS costs is the desire to meet policy objectives – in effect to raise the standard of services. He explained it in managerial terms as better renal services and care in the community. But in setting such policy objectives, the government is responding to demands for different sorts of health care. This can best be summarised as the rising expectations of the health service in a consumer society.

There are two elements in this, of which the first has already been identified as the main factor behind increasing health care budgets in OECD countries. That is the desire of wealthier societies to spend a higher proportion of their income on health. Intuitively, this makes sense. Richer people will spend more on their food and drink; but as the Family Expenditure Survey carried out by the government every year shows, spending on these basic staffs of life does not rise in proportion to income.[20]

For example, households in the bottom tenth of the income distribution devote almost a quarter of their spending to food and non-alcoholic drink; those in the top tenth, less than 15 per cent. While the top tenth spend more than seven times as much as the bottom tenth overall, they spend just

4¼ times as much on food and drink.

To make the point even clearer, there are on average 1.3 people per household in the bottom tenth and 3.2 in the top tenth. Spending per head among the top tenth is greater by 2.9 times than in the bottom tenth; but by only 1.8 times on food.

Richer people have more to spend on the essentials of life such as food, drink and shelter. But it is in other aspects of their lifestyles that their wealth is demonstrated – the amounts spent on entertainment, recreation and luxuries, for example. And while some aspects of health care count as essentials, much of it is optional in the sense of not being necessary to sustain life.

Once the basics of life are taken care of, however, people naturally wish to spend more on raising the quality of their lives – which is where much of what counts as health care comes in. Elective surgery, for example, treats conditions that are not immediately life-threatening and may even be no more than cosmetic. That is not to underestimate the importance of such operations to those who want them. It is merely to understand that they are non-essentials which people choose to have once the essentials of life are taken care of. Thus as societies have more to spend, health care is one thing they like to have more of.

That is the macro-economic side – the demand from society as a whole. There is also a micro-economic element in the form of the health services individuals expect in wealthier societies. With the growth of what is called consumerism, people are less willing to accept 'one size fits all' – the church model of health services which provides the same for everybody. Instead they demand better quality health care services tailored to their particular needs — the garage model of the NHS.

This is, after all, what they get when buying consumer goods. The best producers manage to achieve economies of scale in production while tailoring a range of products to individual needs and markets. Thus there are beers for all tastes, from the traditional draught bitter to the real ales for the cognoscenti and the designer beers for the younger drinkers. Even those who do not regard themselves as well-off are prepared to pay a premium for the pleasure of drinking Mexican or German bottled beer.

The same is also true for services which have undergone a revolution in recent decades to serve their customers better. The most successful private sector organisations try to satisfy their customers' personal preferences, fitting in with their needs and offering services for every taste. They are responsive and open all hours, catering for the needs and lifestyles of an increasingly diverse marketplace.

The provision of travel services is a good example. After the war, holiday camps and UK seaside resorts offered cheap and cheerful holidays for most people, on standard lines. As we learned in Chapter 2, they catered for all classes. Today, some people still like the mass production offered by holiday camps and package tours to popular foreign resorts. But others prefer something more individualistic — self-catering cottages, independent touring abroad and adventurous or educational trips to exotic destinations. New companies have prospered because they have recognised the need for diversity in the industry and offer appropriate holidays.

The National Health Service has lagged behind in recognising that its customers' expectations are changing. Not everyone wants hospital treatment in a ward (though some do); people with busy working lives want to be able to consult doctors at times that are convenient to them; they do not see why operations should not be organised to suit them; and if there is some form of treatment they want which is not available, they do not see why they should be denied it.

One symptom of this is the number of people who consult their general practitioner over the course of a year. Britain is almost certainly a healthier society than ever before, but the proportion of the population seeing a doctor has risen from 66 per cent in 1971–72 to 78 per cent in 1991–92.[21]

The previous government recognised such demands in the Citizen's Charter launched in 1991 by John Major to make essential public services more responsive to their users. Mr Major believed taxpayers using the NHS, state schools and local government services wanted to be treated more like customers than grateful beneficiaries. Each of these public services was therefore required to set quality standards, publicise them and offer redress when services failed to come up to scratch.

The health service section of the Citizen's Charter was the Patient's Charter.[22] As we have already seen, it set targets for service standards such as maximum delays in waiting for treatment and punctuality in appointments between NHS professionals and users. These were no more than the sort of good practice patients had become accustomed to as customers of private sector services.

Over the years, the targets have been raised and new ones added – as for example on mixed-sex wards. Stephen Dorrell, the last Conservative Health Secretary, promised in January 1997 to get rid of this unpopular feature of NHS hospital treatment.[23] The pledge was reinforced in August 1997, when the Labour Health Minister Baroness Jay set a two-year deadline for achieving it.[24]

NHS professionals have often opposed such targets, saying they would add to costs and distort priorities. This is not the experience of the private sector, however. Providing the service customers want – and getting it right first time – has become the key to success.

As Sir Roy Griffiths of Sainsbury's said in response to critics of his plans to beef up NHS management in 1983: 'the hallmarks of truly great organisations in the private sector is that they have placed quality and customer satisfaction first and profit for a long time simply emerged as the by-product of effective services.'[25]

Much of what the Patient's Charter demands is about priorities. It requires those who make decisions in the health service to take patients' preferences into account and not do what they think best or most convenient.

In other services, reorganising around new priorities has led to the use of technology to automate less important parts of the business. In banking, for example, cash machines handle paying in and drawing out to free staff to give financial advice and deal with customers. And once free to focus on the parts of the service they are best at, organisations can contract out the rest to specialists which can do them more cheaply.

This is not to deny that trying to provide a more individually tailored service in the way demanded by the Patient's Charter has no cost implications. The targets for reducing waiting lists challenge the practice adopted by the NHS since its inception of rationing health care by queuing. Reducing cancellations means more spare capacity to deal with the emergencies which lead to operations having to be shelved. And separating the sexes in wards – especially if done in smaller wards which are more like hotels in accommodation standards – bears costs.

That is why there will be upward pressure on health care bills in societies which are becoming better off. It is not because people are living longer or new technology is coming up with the whizzo products of tomorrow's world. It is because people who have more in their pockets want to spend it on the rapidly growing menu of health care services. And they are not prepared to be fobbed off with the sort of rationing celebrated as a communal act of worship when the NHS was founded.

Satisfying rising expectations

The question therefore is what is the best way to reconcile this growing demand for health care from those who are becoming increasingly wealthy, with their reluctance to fund it through a communally financed health service.

The 1991 reforms were designed to create a framework that would get more from less, or at least the same. The internal market would force those working in the NHS to address the demands of patients for a more individual and responsive service. And it would provide the financial disciplines which would allow managers to satisfy such demands from the existing budget.

The then government assumed this could be done without pumping in extra funds because the pre-reform health service lacked the basic disciplines necessary to spend its funds in the most cost-effective way. It was not unreasonable to suppose that once treatments were properly costed and budgets spent to maximise the amount of health care, the rising expectations of patients could be met.

But this neglected the real driver of the increasing cost of the NHS – the desire to spend more on health care simply as a lifestyle decision. Nothing in the reforms created a mechanism that would allow people to increase their spending if that was their choice – and thus the new model health service was bound to disappoint.

6: Rationing is No Answer

Here, then, is the challenge faced by the National Health Service in its 50th year: how to reconcile rising demand in health care with a budget that is unlikely to grow faster than the economy as a whole. In practice, the health service will solve this problem in the same way it has since its inception – by rationing. The difficulty is that the rationing is becoming more obvious to the public which is less likely than ever to accept the consequences.

As we saw in Chapter 2, rationing was built into the NHS at its foundation, in an era when sharing scarce resources was seen as both natural and virtuous. And in the early years, it was understood there was a backlog of treatment from pre-NHS days which inevitably meant delays. But rationing by queuing has remained a central feature of the UK health service, and has reached levels where one in 50 of the population is now on a waiting list.

What Rudolf Klein calls 'rationing by dilution' has also been practised, where the funds have been spread so thinly that some parts of the service are simply inadequate.[1] This way of stretching resources is common throughout the public services. In schools, for example, it leads to large classes where teachers are unable to practise their profession effectively because the priority is to maintain order.

In the health service, long-stay care was subject to such rationing for the first three decades, with patients packed into overcrowded wards under inadequate supervision. This was addressed only after a series of scandals which led Richard Crossman, Labour Social Services Secretary at the end of the 1960s, to discover he was responsible for 'the worst kind of Dickensian, Victorian loony bin'.[2] Today rationing by dilution manifests itself in the poor quality of treatment noted in Chapter 1, which means an NHS hospital stay is rather less salubrious than most people's annual holiday.

Rationing by denial is a third way of reconciling growing demand with limited funds – refusing to cover particular treatments under the NHS. The introduction of kidney dialysis marked the first occasion on which explicit decisions were taken to withhold treatment on grounds of cost.[3] When it became clear in the mid-1960s that it was effective but expensive, the Health Ministry asked the Royal College of Physicians to create an advisory committee of consultants. The outcome was a policy of restricting dialysis to regional centres funded from Whitehall. When home dialysis became possible and kidney transplants were shown to be an option, the number of people treated rose. But as Chapter 1 showed, levels of treatment in the UK remain below those in other European countries – especially for the over-60s.

It is an approach that has been duplicated with other medical developments such as heart and liver transplants. In each case, rationing was obscured by talk of focusing expertise in a few centres while new procedures were proved. But a glance at other countries showed these new treatments to be more widely available overseas – leading to high-profile appeals to raise money for patients to be treated overseas.

However, patients are increasingly reluctant to accept these forms of rationing. Those who can afford it (or get it through their work) vote with their feet by moving into the private sector which now accommodates one in eight of the population. Others can only register their unhappiness with rationing in its various forms through opinion polls.

A short history of NHS rationing

Although the National Health Service has been in the rationing business since its first days, the 'r-word' has remained taboo in official circles. Instead the debate over how to share out the limited health care budget has been conducted in terms of priorities.

The debate first emerged during the 1970s when it became clear the welfare state could not swallow an ever-larger share of the national cake. The 1974–79 Labour government decided to redistribute the health budget from the better-endowed areas to those which were worse off or in greater need. It also increased the funding of the 'Cinderella services', those specialities such as mental health which had been rationed by dilution.

Inevitably this meant less growth in the budget for the better-off areas and specialities. The areas which lost out were London and the south-east, close to the heart of government, the media and the leaders of the medical profession. The impact of this redistribution therefore attracted a disproportionate amount of publicity, fuelling the clamour about underfunding.[4]

Under the Conservative governments of the 1980s, the emphasis switched from inputs – resources – to outputs. Priorities were couched in terms of numbers of particular procedures to be carried out, from open-heart surgery to hip replacements. This is another form of implicit rationing, since doctors and nurses who are busy on heart surgery or hip replacements have less time for other activities such as plastic surgery.

There was a further shift in priorities in the 1990s, with

the white paper *The Health of the Nation* which set targets for the NHS in terms of increasing the number of healthy people.[5] Thus health authorities were enjoined to reduce deaths from coronary heart disease and to minimise the number of suicides. This involved shifting some of the budget from cure to prevention – from acute hospitals to health education.

By the early 1990s, however, the rationing debate had begun to emerge more openly. One reason for this was the 1991 NHS reforms, which dragged the issue of priorities into the open. Before the creation of the internal market, decisions about treatment were taken by practitioners, under the doctrine of clinical autonomy. Everyone in the know recognised that doctors made decisions about whether and how to treat patients which reflected the shortage of resources. But the denial of treatment was carried out through 'individual, fragmented and unrecorded transactions between doctors and patients and/or their relatives', as one analyst put it.[6]

The reforms gave responsibility for deciding what treatments should be available to the purchasers of health care, the health authorities. And as public bodies, they had to be prepared to make their decisions public and justify them. The process was slow to start, since the steady state approach in the first years of the internal market meant most authorities simply contracted for what had been provided before the reforms.

But as health authorities faced mounting demands for treatment and started to focus on priorities, the issue of rationing could no longer be avoided. The first to dip its toe in the water was North East Thames regional health authority. In 1991, it issued guidance on minor surgical procedures which were not to be offered on the NHS unless there was an 'over-riding' need. These included the removal of non-malignant lumps, extraction of wisdom teeth unless they were causing problems, varicose vein operations, *in vitro* fertilisation (IVF) and tattoo removal.[7]

After a public outcry over the exclusions, the authority made clear the procedures could be provided in cases of 'clinical need'. But others followed the lead: a survey by Bath University of the first wave of purchasing plans for 1992–93 found around 10 per cent of the 100-odd authorities planning to deny or limit particular treatments. Tattoo removal was the commonest, followed by IVF and reversal of sterilisation or vasectomy. As well as a variety of cosmetic procedures, the list also included sex change operations and homeopathy.[8]

Nationally, the health service has resisted declaring any form of treatment as outside its remit. Pharmaceuticals, however, are another matter, and in November 1984, the government introduced a 'limited list' of medicines that could not be prescribed under the NHS. This included proprietary cough and cold remedies, antacids, laxatives and mild painkillers – all available as over-the-counter products in chemists.[9] The measure was claimed to save £75 million a year and the list has since been lengthened to include appetite suppressants, pesticides, toiletries, products for diabetics and foodstuffs such as evening primrose oil.[10]

As Tom Sackville, the junior Health Minister who announced the additions in 1993, said: 'The NHS should not be paying for items which have no therapeutic or clinical value . . . Items such as mineral water, cakes, lip salves and face powder cannot be classified as medicines.'[11]

But successive governments have been unwilling to extend this approach to particular forms of treatment, even to procedures which might be seen as having no medical benefits. That approach has been reaffirmed by the new Labour government in its December 1997 white paper, which said the arguments in favour of rationing were not 'convincing'.[12] However, it failed to address the pressures which have led health authorities to begin rationing, implicit or explicit.

And the evidence is that increasing numbers of health authorities are now restricting specific procedures.[13] The range of treatments excluded is also growing, with dilation and curettage for women under 40, various orthodontic treatments and circumcision other than for religious reasons joining tattoo removal and IVF.

Back to basics

The rationale behind the exclusion of some forms of treatment is that there are other health care services the NHS must provide in all circumstances. If resources are limited and outstripped by demand, funding must be preserved for this basic core of treatments because they are, in some sense, essential to the health of the individual.[14]

The health authorities which have been most explicit in rationing appear to have defined the 'core curriculum' by excluding two categories of treatment:

- those for conditions that might be described as self-inflicted – such as tattoo removal
- procedures justified not on medical grounds but on other needs of the patient – as in cosmetic surgery.

In practice, most of these procedures are on the margins of NHS activity and the savings from excluding them likely to be small. But the common ground in both categories is the implication that they are the responsibility of the patient – either because they remedy self-inflicted conditions or are justified on non-medical grounds.

Yet even in these marginal cases, the difficulties in defining a 'core curriculum' are evident. For example, there are perfectly valid medical justifications for tattoo removal. It could be an essential step in getting an individual into paid employment and out of a milieu in which drug abuse is common and a threat to his health.

And with IVF, the cost may be high at an estimated £11,000 per live birth, with a less than even chance of success. But it is the only option for those who cannot be helped by other forms of fertility treatment, and is effective in 40 per cent of women who have three cycles of treatment.

In practice, the decision to include or exclude IVF appears to be as much about power politics as medical evidence. The clinching factor in deciding to fund it appears to be the presence of a consultant locally who argues for it and mobilises opinion in support.[15]

But leaving it to health authorities to make decisions on the core curriculum leads to accusations of 'rationing by postcode' – where treatments are available in one area but not another. This exposes the health service to challenges in the courts over such variation. Whatever the drawbacks of the old centralised NHS, it had at least managed to keep the legal profession largely out of the practice of medicine other than in cases of individual malpractice.[16]

In 1977, for example, patients in the queue for orthopaedic surgery went to court to challenge the Secretary of State over his failure to provide a comprehensive health service. The judge ruled against them, a decision upheld on appeal on the grounds the Health Secretary had done his best 'with the financial resources available to him' and it was not for the courts to question his policies.

Other challenges on denial of treatment have produced similar results over the years, even though the courts have become more willing to overturn government decisions on a wide range of issues. One of the highest profile cases was that of Child B, the 10-year-old girl subsequently named as Jaymee Bowen. In March 1995, her father failed to persuade the Appeal Court to force Cambridge Health Authority to spend £75,000 on further treatment for her leukaemia.

The specialist treating the girl believed it would impose undue suffering with slight chance of success. But her father had found a doctor who was willing to go ahead and wanted the authority to fund the treatment. The court ruled the health authority had acted rationally and fairly and that the funding would not be an effective use of limited resources.[17]

But a recent case indicates how passing rationing decisions on to health authorities can encourage the courts to intervene in the NHS. In July 1997, a multiple sclerosis sufferer succeeded in an action against North Derbyshire health authority over its refusal to fund a course of beta interferon. The authority said the treatment – which costs about £10,000 a patient – was of unproven value and that it had no money to fund it. But a High Court judge said this was 'disingenuous' and ordered the health authority to change its mind. He ruled that North Derbyshire had been less generous than other authorities and had also ignored guidelines on the treatment put out by the NHS Executive.

His judgement therefore did not challenge the overall health budget set in Whitehall but how one district had decided to apply the budget in comparison with others. From the point of view of the patient, this might appear to be little more than a sophistry: something which was previously withheld on grounds of cost can now be extracted by court action. But it opens NHS decisions to legal challenge in a novel way – and one that the government cannot entirely welcome.

Sheltering behind the evidence

Perhaps for these reasons, the move towards excluding particular types of treatment is being accompanied by another trend: the exclusions are becoming less firm. Many health authority purchasing plans now qualify their exclusions by saying they can be carried out if a physician provides persuasive clinical reasons for doing so. Rather than ruling out any particular form of treatment completely, the aim is to cut out treatments in cases where their effectiveness is unproven.

This is what is known as evidence-based medicine – the requirement that treatments be used only where they can be clinically justified. It is an idea whose time has come, since it appears to offer a cost-free form of rationing: if treatment is not effective, withholding it can cause no harm. Indeed, if it does no good, a surgical or pharmaceutical treatment almost certainly carries some risk to the patient and should be stopped. And stopping it is not rationing at all if there is no benefit to the patient's health.

Some have seen evidence-based medicine as making a significant contribution to bridging the health service's funding gap – among them, Sir Michael Peckham, the NHS's first research director. During his time in Whitehall, he backed a heavyweight research programme into clinical effectiveness and initiatives to disseminate information to clinicians. When Sir Michael departed from the post in January 1996, he said that evidence-based medicine could release at least £1 billion a year for improved patient care by cutting out unnecessary treatments.[18]

This view now has weighty backing from the new Labour government. Its December 1997 white paper commits the NHS to 'reducing inappropriate treatments' and increasing 'provision of treatments proven to bring benefits'.[19] It promises a new National Institute for Clinical Excellence to produce and disseminate guidelines on best practice in terms of 'clinical and cost-effectiveness' [sic].[20]

There are certainly plenty of examples to back up the view that there are savings to be made from excluding ineffective procedures – among them the insertion of grommets in children's ears.[21] This is a treatment for glue ear, the condition behind The War of Jennifer's Ear discussed in Chapter 3. Caused by a viscous substance in the middle ear, it affects the hearing of about 5 per cent of children between two and four. It is distressing for the children concerned and perhaps more so for their anxious parents.

Inserting the grommets – at an approximate cost of £300 each – often leads to improved hearing, though the condition may still recur. At the beginning of the 1990s, the NHS found itself spending more than £30 million a year on inserting grommets in children's ears. It was the eighth most common operation in 1992–93 and ate up a large proportion of the budget for hospital ear, nose and throat departments.

Despite the operation's apparent efficacy, however, the research evidence is that it is unnecessary in most cases. If left alone, glue ear usually clears up of its own accord and without too much delay – within three months in about half the cases. Grommet insertion is therefore often now identified in purchasing plans as a procedure for more selective use, with guidelines for alternative approaches such as 'watchful waiting' and regular hearing tests.

Such an approach clearly has attractions beyond saving money. If properly handled, watchful waiting is greatly preferable in most parents' eyes to an operation on their child. And from the child's point of view, it eliminates the need for a form of treatment which – like all operations – carries its own risks.

However, it is not always so simple. For one thing, agreement on what is effective in medicine is harder to reach than you might think. It is rather like the observation made by David Ogilvy, the advertising guru, that half the money spent on advertising is wasted: the problem is we don't know which half.

A surprisingly small proportion of treatments has been demonstrated to be effective under the sort of testing scientists would regard as rigorous. This does not necessarily mean the others are ineffective: they may not have been tested, or they may be only partly effective. But if they work for some people or they do no harm and ameliorate suffering, then they may have value.

Clearly it is hard to defend inserting grommets in a child's ear when waiting a few weeks might lead to a complete cure. But the prescription of a placebo can be the prelude to a cure – if only because it contributes to the patient's well-being in other ways. Equally, some forms of alternative medicine may be effective for some people precisely because they address non-medical concerns which undermine good health.

It is even more difficult to insist on a rigorous testing pro-gramme before use in the case of cures for fatal conditions or those that severely disable. The case of beta interferon, re-ferred to above, is an example: health authorities which refuse to fund it do so because they believe it has not been demonstrably proved effective. A multiple sclerosis patient will understandably feel that if there appears to be a chance of success, it is worth trying.

Even more heart-breaking decisions have had to be made in the case of HIV patients. Those in advanced stages of AIDS are often prepared to be human guinea pigs if new drugs or cocktails of drugs appear promising. When the chances of survival or remission are as low as they can be in such cases, demanding double blind tests seems callous in the extreme.

Can treatment be cost-effective?

If particular treatments cannot be excluded completely, the question is then whether there are alternative criteria to allow the clinician to make decisions about treatment when resources are limited. One answer is cost-benefit analysis – comparing the benefits of one treatment against those of an-other and focusing on the one that produces the greatest 'health gain' per pound spent. However, finding a measure of cost-effectiveness that would command widespread support has largely defeated those who support this approach.

The idea that the NHS should concentrate on remedies with the greatest chance of success has great intuitive appeal. Physicians have long made decisions in their everyday practice on a rough and ready cost-benefit basis – cost being interpreted in its widest sense. It is always a matter of fine judgement about when the struggle to prolong life should cease, usually in the interests of the patient.

Sometimes cruder rules of thumb emerge which are implicit in rationing decisions – for example that certain operations will not normally be performed on people over a certain age. Opinion polls suggest some public support for using age as a criterion for rationing, no doubt based on the view that older people have had a 'good innings'.[22] But this sort of crude rationing by age could be justified only if age is a sure-fire indicator of ability to benefit – if older people have much less chance of surviving a treatment, for example. The Queen Mother's hip replacement shows it is hard to be categorical in such matters: there are people even in their 90s who can expect to live long enough to make worthwhile those procedures routinely denied to the elderly.

In other cases, the implicit judgement is that the effort is better devoted to someone with more of their life ahead of them. This would appear to be the justification in the case of kidney dialysis, and other studies have found similar judgements in stroke units and transplant units.

But such decisions have become explicit following the 1991 reforms. Health authorities must explain their priorities in purchasing health care; trusts must explain how they will allocate particular budgets between the cases referred to them by general practitioners. The issue of rationing by age was one of the first to emerge after the 1991 reforms were launched.

In April 1994, the BBC Radio 4 *Today* programme featured a 73-year-old man denied physiotherapy by a hospital because he was over 65 – a policy that had been explained to local GPs in a letter. The director of the physiotherapy unit was quoted as saying 'there must be some cut-off point', and because people below 65 would be more likely to be in work they needed to get better quickly.[23] The resulting outcry forced the then Health Secretary Virginia Bottomley to rule it was unacceptable for the NHS to make decisions other than on clinical need. 'There are no exceptions to this rule, whatever the age of the patient,' she said.[24]

There is also the question of lifestyle, and how it impinges on the likelihood of recovery. In 1993, Harry Elphick, a heavy smoker from Manchester, was denied treatment for a heart condition because he refused to give up smoking. Mr Elphick pointed out he had paid more than his fair share of tax as a smoker and was entitled to treatment. The clinicians argued the operation would have been ineffective; critics said the doctors were making a judgement on a lifestyle they disapproved of. Mr Elphick died later that year, prompting Mrs Bottomley to issue a further ukase reminding doctors that clinical need was the only concern.[25]

Many people find the idea that treatment should be focused on those who are most likely to benefit from it more persuasive when a condition can be attributed to behaviour thought foolish or dangerous by informed opinion – whether it be smoking, drinking, drug abuse or sexual promiscuity. But even if doctors obey Mrs Bottomley's prescription and stick to clinical need, there will be choices to make between cases with greatly differing chances of success.

For example, we saw earlier that those who oppose offering IVF on the NHS often cite its cost in comparison with other forms of treatment. If the comparison is with other forms of infertility treatment, it is a false one, however: IVF is a way of treating people for whom the alternatives will not work.

But the cost of one cycle of IVF can instead be compared with other forms of treatment. One health authority points out that a new hip can be bought for one cycle of IVF treatment – which has only a one in four chance of success.[26] This is very unsatisfactory however: it would be hard to reach agreement on the different benefits from this same cost – a baby that could not otherwise be born versus an improvement in the quality of life for perhaps many years.

One tool for comparing the benefits from different types of treatment is the Quality-Adjusted Life Year, or QALY. Devised in the 1970s, this measures the cost of delivering a year of life at some defined level of quality – in other words giving more weight to treatments which fully restore patients than those that leave them below par. This can lead on to comparing various treatment options to see which is the 'best buy'.[27]

Thus one 1990 study found the cost per QALY for cholesterol testing and treatment by diet for adults aged 40 to 69 in danger of coronary heart disease was £220. The cost per

QALY if the patient ended up needing an operation was much higher: £2,090 for a coronary artery bypass graft for a patient with severe angina, £7,480 for a heart transplant and £18,830 for a bypass in a case of moderate angina. Thus prevention was clearly much better value for money than cure.

This approach offers a rational basis for making rationing decisions. Treatments can be ranked in terms of QALYs with greater priority given to those further up the list. And it has been adopted by a significant minority of health authorities: a survey carried out by the King's Fund Institute in 1992 found a fifth using QALY evidence to assist decision-making. Almost as many unequivocally planned to do so.[28] The Department of Health is encouraging work on the concept.

But there are both technical and practical difficulties in using this approach in a hard and fast way.[29] Technically, there are problems in calculating QALYs, since the benefits of particular forms of treatment may be sensitive to small changes in assumptions. For example, the people currently treated may be those most likely to benefit, so extending the treatment to others may produce fewer QALYs per case. Equally, the success rate of an operation may be lower if it is used more widely. And the comparisons may rely on some broad-brush assumptions about the relative weight of, say, one year of robust health with, say, three years of greatly improved mobility.

The practical difficulties of a cost-benefit analysis lie more in the public realm, where there are deeply rooted human values that defy a rationalist approach. How, for example, can it be applied to groups such as the mentally handicapped? Is it possible to compare the benefits of a course of drugs for an acute schizophrenic with those of a hip replacement operation or a life-saving operation? And who decides the weighting to give a year of severely disabled life? A disabled person might assess it rather differently than a member of the general public. There is value even in years of incapacity – as can be seen from the experience of Christy Brown, the cerebral palsy sufferer whose book *My Left Foot* became an award-winning film that touched millions.[30]

At a more popular level, the QALY-type approach just does not command support – as the MORI poll carried out for the Social Market Foundation in summer 1997 indicated. Those surveyed were asked to choose between cancer treatment for a 45-year-old with two dependent children and a hip operation for a 75-year-old. The cancer treatment had only a one in ten chance of giving the patient a fulfilling life of more than a year while the hip operation would give up to 10 years' dramatic improvement in the older patient's life.[31] Yet 63 per cent wanted priority given to the cancer patient – the family commitment clearly outweighing cost-effectiveness in the public mind.

The QALY would also appear to discriminate against the elderly, who have less to gain in terms of years of life than younger people. It would make it harder to get very expensive forms of treatment, including those needed by some extremely ill people who could be fully restored to health. And it might imply giving priority to people who were more likely to make a full recovery – because they were non-smokers, for example, or not overweight, or simply middle-class folk whose diet and lifestyle were healthier.[32]

A further complication is that most people give greater

priority to measures that save lives than to those designed to improve the quality of life.[33] Breast cancer screening costs £5,780 per QALY, for example, and would buy five hip replacements. But many people would see it as more important to discover a case of breast cancer in time to treat it than to replace several dozen hip joints.

And saving a particular life always appears more attractive than spending money to reduce deaths at some time in the future in the population as a whole. That is why it is hard to divert resources from high-profile techniques such as heart transplants to what is undoubtedly a much more effective approach to heart disease: paying general practitioners to give advice about giving up smoking.

None of this is to deny that cost-benefit analysis has something to add to the process of setting priorities in health care. It is another tool for stimulating public debate over the best use of public funds. And it is a discipline that should be used to review priorities and challenge established ways of doing things. But it is unlikely to shift popular opinion on the merits of treating elderly people or heavy smokers – however convincing the figures.

In other words, if cost-benefit analysis is to be used as a tool for setting priorities, it must remain at the level of generalities. There will always be the fabled smoker who lives until 98 while smoking 40 untipped cigarettes a day, while other people who have never touched the weed are carried off at half the age by heart attacks.

The aggregates involved in calculating QALYs can help in comparing different approaches, or in evaluating the merits of preventive measures against cleaning up the mess later. But they cannot be translated into individual decisions over treatment.

Searching for the core

The search for a formula that would restrict public funding to core health care services is not a uniquely British phenomenon. High-profile attempts to reach a public consensus on priorities have taken place elsewhere, including the Netherlands, New Zealand and Sweden as well as various parts of the United States.

In America, the most interesting rationing exercise has been in the state of Oregon. It mounted lengthy consultations to draw up a priority list for around 700 treatments offered under Medicaid, the publicly funded programme for people below retirement age who have no health insurance.[34]

The first step was to establish community views on priorities – preventative medicine versus life-saving operations, for example – and values such as equity and quality of life. A commission used this information plus a certain amount of cost-benefit analysis to rank the treatments. Their measure was the DALY – the disability-adjusted life year – which gives greater weight than the DALY to extra years of lower quality. Eventually agreement was reached on retaining 565 treatments, a saving which allowed the state to extend Medicaid coverage to people previously excluded because their income was too high to qualify.

Successful though the Oregon exercise appears, it is not without its critics. The process was not quite as systematic as planned, for example. The initial rankings produced some odd results, including rating cosmetic breast surgery higher than treatment for an open thigh fracture. They were therefore adjusted to make them look more reasonable and acceptable.[35]

Despite taking five years to complete, the exercise attracted very little public involvement. Only just over a thousand people attended the meetings to establish community views, two-thirds of them health care workers. Fewer than 5 per cent were recipients of Medicaid.[36]

The exercise seems to have worked for Oregon – perhaps because it produced tangible benefits in terms of wider coverage of the population. But an approach designed for a sparsely populated, largely rural state has yet to be applied elsewhere in America. And it is of limited relevance in countries such as the UK where rationing must involve taking something away from a population that believes it has universal coverage from its health service.

Other overseas experiences in countries with health services more like that of the UK have been less satisfactory in setting priorities for rationing. In the Netherlands, for example, the task was performed by the Dunning Committee, created in 1990 to advise on a basic package of health care benefits for everyone. It made good headway by establishing four criteria:[37]

- the care should be necessary from the community's point of view
- it must be shown to be effective
- it must be efficient
- it could not be left to individuals to pay for themselves.

The committee showed how these principles might be

applied in practice.[38] *In vitro* fertilisation, for example, failed the necessity test – childlessness posed no danger to the community, it said, and did not stop the individual functioning normally in Dutch society. Homeopathy failed on effectiveness and efficiency and was, in any case, cheap enough for the patient to pay the bills. Dental care was also affordable by the patient and could be excluded.

But the committee said the decision on what to exclude was ultimately a political one. Perhaps not surprisingly, Dutch politicians have largely decided to duck the issue. Instead the emphasis is now on cutting out the waste of treatments used in inappropriate situations. As in the UK, the decision has been passed to the individual clinician, and the burden placed on evidence-based medicine.

In New Zealand, a national advisory committee set up in 1992 to give continuing advice on the core health service almost immediately decided to reject blanket exclusions.[39] It said even the least efficacious treatments could be justified medically in some circumstances – as in the example of tattoo-removal given earlier. Instead it decided to work with the medical profession to develop criteria such as cost-effectiveness in deciding priorities, and to test their acceptability against public opinion. Again, the consequence is that the decision is left ultimately with the clinician.

A Swedish parliamentary commission created to set priorities went one step further in its 1995 report by relegating cost-effectiveness behind two other principles:[40]

- human dignity – that all should be treated equally irrespective of their personal characteristics or status in the community

- need and solidarity – resources should go to those needing them the most, such as the mentally ill who deserve special consideration.

Only after these two principles have been considered should cost-effectiveness come into play, the commission decided. Thus it would never be right to lay down general rules about a particular form of treatment on a cost basis – money should be a consideration only when choosing between options for treating a particular patient. In other words, it should all be left to the clinician.

Is scarcity inevitable?

So in almost every case, attempting to curb the freedom of clinicians by rationing health care comes full circle. The process starts by trying to exclude particular treatments, but falters when it comes to difficult cases. It slips into the idea that particular procedures should be subject to closer checks to make sure they are appropriate and/or effective. Finally, it ends up throwing the responsibility for making the decisions back to the clinician in the light of the individual patient's needs.

We are thus back where we started, with the doctor making opaque decisions in the privacy of the consulting room or operating theatre. The practice of medicine is the application of medical knowledge to particular patients in the light of their circumstances. The only requirement is that two cases in identical need – whatever that means – be treated identically and preferably by ways that are proven to work.

The NHS has succeeded in bridging the gap between supply and demand since its inception by concealed rationing –

queuing, dilution and denial dressed up in clinical justifications. But the growing demands of patients in a consumerist
age are widening the gap and making it impossible to continue this approach.

Hence the search for a set of explicit principles to ration
the health care budget fairly. That search fails because the
needs of individual patients are so different. The only rationing principles acceptable to public opinion add up to little more than exhorting physicians not to waste money.

However, the debate over rationing succeeds in obscuring
the more important issue in health care: why there is a gap
between supply and demand. To phrase the question differently, is the scarcity of the post-war years which gave birth to
the NHS an inevitable part of the landscape 50 years later? If
it is, then rationing is here to stay, and we had better find
some way of agreeing on how it should be done.

A first answer is that it would be crazy were that to be
true. We have already established that health care is something people want more of as they become wealthier – and
they can afford to spend more on it. Our present system of
financing the health service through taxation makes it very
hard to spend the extra, for several reasons. One is that the
health budget all goes into a common pot, so people who
want to spend more on themselves cannot be sure they will
benefit from additional contributions. Another is the generalised loss of faith in public institutions – based on experience – which means taxpayers do not believe that higher
taxes will inevitably produce better services. Finally, not
everyone will want to spend more on health – and those
who do not should be free to make that choice.

The second answer is to search for alternative ways to bridge the gap between supply and demand in health care – the issue which will be explored in the next chapter. But the debate over rationing is at least useful in the question it asks over what is appropriate for a publicly funded health service to offer. We shall return to this issue in Chapter 9.

7: The Real Crisis in the NHS

Ask anyone what the problem of the National Health Service is and the answer is likely to be shortage of money. Ask where the additional money should come from, and the answer will almost equally likely be from taxation. A MORI opinion poll in summer 1997 found three-quarters of adults thought the NHS was underfunded and 55 per cent wanted taxes to be raised to remedy the situation.[1] Other polls – including the British Social Attitudes survey discussed in Chapter 1 – find similar results.

Certainly there appears to be a strong case for saying Britain needs to spend more on health care. Figures produced by the Organisation for Economic Co-operation and Development, in Table 7.1, show the UK towards the bottom of the league table in spending on health services as a percentage of gross domestic product.

The cash figures make the UK's spending look even smaller, at about half the level per head of that in France and Germany. But these figures are based on exchange rates between the currencies of the various countries, which are subject to the vagaries of the foreign exchange markets. Most economists prefer to make comparisons in terms of purchasing power parities – exchange rates based on the value of currencies in terms of what they can buy.

A simple example would be *The Economist's* Big Mac index, which readjusts exchange rates to make a Big Mac hamburger cost the same in every country. The most recent survey by the magazine showed the exchange rate between the dollar and sterling should be £1 = $1.34 if a Big Mac was to cost the same in the UK as in America. On the day of the survey, 7 April 1997, the actual exchange rate was £1 = $1.63

– suggesting the official exchange rate was 22 per cent over-valued.[2]

Table 7.1
Health spending in selected OECD countries, 1994

Country	% of GDP	£ per capita
United States	14.3	2,285
Canada	9.8	1,182
France	9.7	1,449
Austria	9.7	1,559
Switzerland	9.6	2,286
Germany	9.5	1,552
Netherlands	8.8	1,249
Finland	8.3	1,041
Italy	8.3	967
Belgium	8.2	1,199
Ireland	7.9	746
Sweden	7.7	1,126
Portugal	7.6	435
Spain	7.3	592
UK	**6.9**	**787**
Denmark	6.6	1,214
Greece	5.2	315
OECD average	**7.9**	**1,101**
EU (15) average	**7.8**	**1,037**

Source: Office of Health Economics, *Compendium of Health Statistics*, 1997, Tables 2.2, 2.3.

The OECD carries out some much more sophisticated surveys to calculate purchasing power parities, the results of
which are in Table 7.2. This shows that health spending per
head is correlated with GDP per head – a few outliers such as

Table 7.2
Health spending compared in terms of buying power, 1995

US dollars, converted at purchasing power parities

Country	GDP per head	Health spending per head
United States	26,438	3,701
Switzerland	24,809	2,412
Denmark	21,529	1,368
Canada	21,031	2,049
Belgium	20,792	1,665
Austria	20,772	1,634
Germany	20,497	2,134
France	19,939	1,956
Netherlands	19,782	1,728
Italy	19,464	1,507
Sweden	18,673	1,360
Finland	17,788	1,373
UK	**17,756**	**1,246**
Ireland	17,228	1,106
Spain	14,226	1,075
Portugal	12,457	1,035
Greece	12,174	703

Source: British Medical Association, *Options for Funding Healthcare*, 1997,
Table 2.

Denmark apart. Measured in this way, the UK's expenditure on health is not so different to those of countries with a similar GDP per head such as Sweden, Finland and Ireland.

The clear message from Table 7.2 is that the higher the GDP per head, the higher the spending on health care – adding further force to the contention that people in Britain will want to spend more on their health as they become wealthier.

Good value for money?

Given such figures, the argument can be made that the NHS is an efficient way of getting a reasonable health service at an affordable cost. Judged by any of the broad measures of health such as life expectancy, infant mortality and the like, the UK health service stands comparison with most other countries. And it can be argued that spending more will not necessarily produce better health. The United States spends almost twice as much as the UK on health care, but has markedly higher infant mortality rates, for example.

For most Americans, of course, the quality of health care they enjoy is rather higher than that on offer in the UK. The delays in receiving treatment in the NHS and the shabby conditions of many hospitals and surgeries appal visitors from across the Atlantic. And while the American approach has much that is wrong about it, it manages to do better by some measures. It is, for example, easier to get kidney dialysis in the free-market US health system than in the UK – as one historian of the NHS points out:

Ironically the NHS, with its strong commitment to

equality, has allowed less egalitarian access to dialysis machines than the market-oriented American system, which historically has had a relatively low commitment to equality of access to care. In the case of chronic renal dialysis, 'the result of rationing is clearly death'.[3]

Such observations do not make the US health care system better, but they should lead us to look a little more critically at the shortcomings of the NHS. The American approach is good at dolloping out large amounts of jam on to the toast – giving more to some people than they really want or need, but leaving some bits uncovered. The NHS is more like Marmite, spread thinly but equally across the piece. But anyone who wants more than Marmite has to join the queue for jam, with no guarantee they will get it. Once again, Rudolf Klein sums it up pithily: 'The pathology of the American health care system . . . is the risk of overtreatment. Conversely, the pathology of the NHS is the risk of undertreatment.'[4]

Health economists might rejoice at the ability of the NHS to restrain health care spending, but the real question is why that should be seen as virtuous. Clearly there is unsatisfied demand at the moment, as the swiftly lengthening waiting lists indicate. And as some of the stories in Chapter 1 suggest, what is on offer now is well below the standards expected in other parts of life.

In any case, there is nothing wrong with a society spending more on health care – so long as it is what people want, having thought about the alternatives they are forgoing by so doing. As noted in Chapter 5, wealthier societies are likely to spend a higher proportion of their income on health services. There are also benefits for the economy in a buoyant health care sector: it is labour-intensive, the jobs are less influenced by the economic cycle and it is less exposed to international competition than the production of traded goods or services.[5]

The reason why there is public interest in restraining health care expenditure is that the NHS is publicly funded. The cost of the nation's food bill, the amount it spends on housing or travel, the level of demand for cinema tickets, computer games or cable television – none of these are matters for public concern. No one suggests it would be good for the country to rein in the rise in spending on home computers, or that the share of GDP spent on tourism should be capped. The reason is that these are not publicly funded activities, straining the public purse. The decisions about how much to spend are in the hands of individual consumers.

There are, in fact, reasonable cases to be made for restraining some of these other forms of spending. Economists could point out that spending less on overseas travel and more on health care would boost UK employment and reduce the balance of payments deficit. Nutritionists would argue that spending less on junk food would improve the nation's health and reduce the cost of handling the consequences of a bad diet. But a politician or economist who advanced such arguments would get short shrift from the public and enjoy five minutes of media abuse for 'nannying'.

Yet holding back the growth in health care spending is widely seen as an important aim of public policy – whatever the shortcomings of the NHS. Indeed, most of the countries which belong to the Organisation for Economic Co-operation and Development have publicly funded health services which they are struggling to contain. So too are the governments in countries where health services are provided by private insurers – since the state usually looks after those who cannot afford to pay insurance premiums, it has an interest in holding down its share of the overall bill.

The only reason the state feels it needs to curb health spending is the fiscal burden on individuals and employers when health care is publicly funded. Voters say they would be prepared to pay more in taxes to have better health services – but are unwilling to vote for parties that promise to put up taxes to do just that. Therefore the role of the NHS is to hold back growth in health care spending when demand is increasing and funding rising more slowly.

If people spent their own money in the health service, no one would feel reducing the total spend was an important issue. There are good reasons why people cannot be expected to spend their own money to provide for *all* their health care needs, which we will look at in the next chapter. But if people want to spend more on health services and are unwilling to do it collectively through the NHS, then the only alternative is to allow them to spend more themselves.

Thinking the unthinkable

In fact, the UK is rather different from other western European countries in the extent to which it relies on public funding for health care. As Table 7.3 shows, most of our European partners draw a larger share of the finance for their health services from private funding.

Table 7.3
**Share of health spending from public and private sources,
1994**

Country	% of GDP on public health spending	% of GDP on private health spending	Public spending as % of total health bill
France	7.6	2.1	78.4
Belgium	7.2	1.0	87.9
Canada	7.0	2.8	71.8
Germany	7.0	2.5	73.5
Switzerland	6.9	2.7	71.8
Netherlands	6.9	1.9	77.6
Sweden	6.4	1.3	83.4
United States	6.3	8.0	44.3
Austria	6.2	3.5	63.4
Finland	6.2	2.1	75.2
Ireland	6.0	1.9	76.0
Italy	5.9	2.4	70.6
UK	**5.8**	**1.1**	**84.1**
Spain	5.7	1.6	78.6
Denmark	5.4	1.2	83.0
Greece	3.5[*]	1.7	75.8

[*] 1993 figure
Source: Office of Health Economics, *Compendium of Health Statistics*,
1997, Tables 2.5, 2.9, 2.24.

One country where people are expected to make a contribution towards their health care is – perhaps surprisingly –
Sweden, the epitome of European social democracy. Swedes

pay a charge of between £10 and £20 to see a doctor, whether in a health centre or at a hospital. The level of fees is set by the counties which administer their health service, up to a maximum set by the government of £20 a visit and £160 per patient per year. There are also hospital in-patient fees at a modest rate of around £5 a day, waived for children under 16.[6]

Most attempts to compare Sweden with other countries show it has greater equality in health outcomes than the UK – in spite of these charges.[7] Indeed, most European countries expect patients to pay to see a doctor, even if the charge is waived or subsequently refunded for those on low incomes.

The Netherlands is going furthest in its ambitious health care reform, which will require employees to pay an annual fee in the form of a flat-rate insurance premium that covers about 10 per cent of health expenditure.[8] Again, Dutch health inequalities are less than those of the British.

One further – somewhat exceptional – case needs also to be considered in thinking about payments: that of Switzerland. Unique in western Europe, the Swiss have an entirely private health insurance system. On the standard measures of health equality, Switzerland comes out ahead of the UK (and many other European countries). One analyst sums up the relationship between paying and health inequality as follows:

> In terms of differences in the delivery of health care, Britain and Spain emerge poorly, while Denmark and Switzerland have the least inequity. Thus there appears to be inequity favouring the rich in some countries where public cover is universal and comprehensive, notably

Spain and Britain. Conversely, health care systems that do not have universal and comprehensive public cover are not necessarily those with the highest degree of inequality. Indeed, inequity appears to be less in countries such as the Netherlands (where cover is income-related) and in Switzerland (where public cover is virtually non-existent).[9]

So it is not the experience of other European countries that expecting a private contribution for health services – of itself – leads to greater inequality than in the UK. What, then, are the theoretical arguments against wider use of charges?

The case for and against charging

Suggesting that people should spend some of their own money on health care can be relied on to produce an outcry. The protests have two elements: first, since people are already paying for the NHS through their taxes, they should not be required to spend more; second, it would be unfair, because some people would not be able to afford to pay more and thus end up with inferior services.[10]

The first is easily disposed of. We are already paying as much for the NHS through taxation as we seem prepared to pay – and it is not enough. The last Conservative government did its best to squeeze more bang for each buck spent on the health service but, as we have seen, did little to satisfy de-mand. Extra bucks need to come from somewhere and al-lowing patients to pay some of the cost is one way of generating that additional funding.

The second objection – on grounds of fairness – is harder to deal with. Clearly if people are required to top up what is offered by the NHS, some will be able to afford to pay more than others. Most people instinctively do not want to live in a country where some can afford essential health care and others can not. As the government's December 1997 white paper reminds us, 'Two-thirds [of people in the British Social Attitudes survey] believe that health care should be available to all on the basis of need, not ability to pay.'[11] One way to avoid that is to have a commonly funded health service to which all contribute and from which all get the same treatment – irrespective of need.

Some of the assumptions of this argument are, however, open to challenge. If charging is introduced into the health service, the government can protect low-income patients by waiving their charges or reimbursing them, as happens in other European countries. A health service with charges can still effectively present itself to the patient as free at the point of use – it does not have to involve credit checks before treatment is given.

And it is possible to distinguish essential health care such as life-saving operations from procedures which are less essential – if equally important to particular individuals. Anyone involved in a car accident or who is suffering a heart attack needs the same immediate treatment, and should get it. But there will be choices to be made in the subsequent treatment – for example, over the sort of accommodation or the timing of therapy. If some people are willing to spend their money to exercise choice in such circumstances, it does not inevitably leave those who cannot afford to make such choices worse off in health terms.

Finally, the current NHS model offering universal health service free at the point of use is failing to deliver. As we have seen in earlier chapters, it is proving unable to provide treatment to all irrespective of need. Meanwhile, the one in nine people who are covered by private health insurance are already offered better treatment than those who rely on the health service. And as we shall see in Chapter 9, even the free service fails to reach those who need it.

Encouraging people to chip in some extra contribution above what they are prepared to pay through their taxes might reduce this inequality by bringing extra resources into the NHS. But charging might also bring additional benefits, not least in deterring people from wasting the scarce time of doctors, nurses and other health professionals. A service that is free is often one which is not valued, and may be abused. Most people working in the health service know of cases of frivolous demands – and of demands that reflect non-medical needs such as isolation, loneliness and mental ill-health.

General practitioners can reel off the names of their 'frequent attenders', the 10–20 per cent of patients who occupy 80 per cent of their time. Some of these have chronic conditions that force them to attend regularly, but many others do not. Often it is enough to point out to the latter that they are frequent attenders – they had simply never realised and resolve to be less demanding. But a charge would invite everyone using the health service to think twice about consuming a scarce resource.

A further attraction of charging would be if it discouraged behaviour that is injurious to health. Many health professionals who disagreed with the decision to deny Harry El-phick treatment because he would not stop smoking, nonetheless felt a pang of irritation that such bad cases should become the focus of attention. At present, patients have no incentive to look after their health since there is no direct financial penalty when it breaks down. In many other walks of life, charges encourage people to take steps to avoid incurring them – whether it is taking basic security precautions to reduce insurance premiums or parking legally to avoid the attentions of traffic wardens.

Economists would add another attraction in charging: that it tells us about patients' preferences. A free service may be consumed simply because it is free: when British Rail offered free travel for a day to pensioners, many took up the offer for pointless journeys that filled trains and crowded out paying passengers. If there is a charge that reflects the cost of a service, people may decide not to use it and spend the money on something else.

The classic example is school dinners, which were once heavily subsidised and of indifferent quality. When the subsidy fell and the charge rose, parents and children switched to sandwiches, and school meal organisers were forced to provide more of the sort of food the children wanted.[12] In the health service, all sorts of tests may be carried out if there is no charge, but the patient might be more questioning if he or she had to pay for them.

Finally, paying for something – rather than getting it as an act of charity – may empower the users. They will demand higher standards and seek to be treated as a customer rather than a supplicant. The NHS would probably be a more effective organisation if its patients did not feel grateful for whatever service they get – as suggested by the *Which?* survey mentioned in Chapter 1.

But health care has significant differences in relation to other forms of spending which mean charges might not produce such benefits. Chief among these differences is what economists call an 'information asymmetry': patients do not have the knowledge about medicine to act like consumers. That is why we concede to the medical profession decisions over which treatment is necessary, what kind to go for and its duration. We appoint the doctor as our agent, to choose the right course of action for us in circumstances where we have little option but to accept the advice given. For this reason, much of medicine is supply-led. It is often not the patient who demands an expensive or complex form of treatment; it is the doctor who recommends it.[13] The idea that the patient can exercise control over the health service or force it to be more efficient is fanciful.

It is also fanciful to expect charges for health care to lead to startling improvements in healthy behaviour. The overwhelming evidence about the impact of smoking on health has had little effect on the 38 per cent of the population who still smoke – few of whom can doubt that it is injurious to their health. Nor has the disincentive of hefty taxes on tobacco done the trick. Even in such a well-established cause and effect, smokers cannot connect a change in their behaviour now – which would have large financial benefits – with an improvement in health later.

While charges might deter timewasters, they could also stop people going to the doctor when it would be in their interests to do so. If patients wait until it is clear something is wrong with them, their treatment could be far costlier – and the consequences of the condition much more serious. Imposing charges for seeing a doctor could end up being an expensive mistake if it led to more emergency admissions to hospitals.

Finally, even those of us who could afford to pay more for health services might lose out if others cannot. Health is a classic public good: we all have an interest in reducing the incidence of illness – AIDS, for example, pays no respect to class. If publicly funded health care is seen as inferior to the health services enjoyed by those who pay, it could find it harder to reach patients – even if the reality is that it is no worse. In other words, non-payers would feel stigmatised, and we might all end up worse off if we have to deal with the consequences of their resulting ill-health.

None of these factors rules out asking patients to pay for some of their treatment or to play a more active role in the process. They are adverse consequences which need to be addressed if people are to pay for more of their health care – and we will return to them in Chapter 9. But they suggest that one set of expectations over the introduction of charges might be unrealistic. That is the idea that if patients were allowed to pay to some degree for their treatment, a full-blown market could emerge in which medical services are bought by patients acting as consumers in the way they do in other walks of life.

Most patients will continue to rely on their doctor for advice, and will want to have whatever treatment he or she recommends. What paying might offer is some extra funds for the NHS, allowing patients to choose to spend more than they are prepared to pay currently through their taxes. It could curb the waste of resources that every doctor knows happens – whether it be patients requesting unnecessary appointments with GPs or doctors recommending treatments of doubtful value. And it could offer patients some choices about their treatment, revealing their preferences on how their health care is delivered.

The NHS experience

Whatever the advantages, charging is antithetical to the very nature of the National Health Service, which was designed to provide universal health care free at the point of use. That is what it did for the first three years, with the financial consequences outlined in Chapter 2. But despite the furore over the introduction of charges for teeth and spectacles in 1951, charges have always played a minor role in the health service – never providing much more than 5 per cent of its funds. Repeated attempts by the Treasury to introduce a greater degree of charging have largely foundered – even under the redoubtable Margaret Thatcher.[14] After 18 years of a government frequently accused of wanting to privatise the health service, patient payments – charges at the point of use – accounted for just 2.3 per cent of NHS income in 1996. Prescription charges raised £421 million, dental charges £515 million and hospital charges £50 million.[15]

In most cases, decisions to introduce or increase charging have been as much about economic policy as about health issues. The charges that forced Bevan's resignation, for example, were to help finance rearmament during the Korean war. When the Conservatives doubled prescription charges in 1956, it was a sop to the private sector to demonstrate Treasury willingness to make sacrifices in the public sector. And the reintroduction of prescription charges in 1968 was said by Roy Jenkins, the then Chancellor, to be 'disproportionately valuable on account of the impression it makes on bankers'. A similar argument was used by the 1974 Labour government when it raised charges in 1976 as part of the package of measures at the time of the International Monetary Fund loan.[16]

Charges were steadily increased throughout Mrs Thatcher's terms in office, peaking at 4.5 per cent of NHS income in 1989–90. Her governments raised dental charges to cover nearly 40 per cent of costs in the mid-1980s, though the figure has since dropped back to 30 per cent. NHS spectacles were replaced by vouchers for those on low incomes and in 1988, free eye tests were abolished for most people. Prescription charges were raised from 45p an item in 1979 to £3.05 in 1990 (and have since risen to £5.65). In contrast to earlier increases in charges, however, the aim was to ease pressure on the health budget by raising revenue and deterring waste.

Yet as noted above, the contribution made by charges has dropped since Mrs Thatcher's time. Prescription charges cover less than 10 per cent of the NHS drugs bill, and five out of six prescriptions are to people who are exempt from paying. This is because so many groups are exempt: men over 65 and women over 60; children under 19 and still in full-time education; expectant mothers and those with a child under 12 months; people on means-tested benefits or slightly above the threshold; and people with certain chronic ailments such as diabetes. The proportion of prescription items exempt from the charge has risen steadily from 65 per cent in 1979 to 84 per cent in 1995–96.[17]

These figures show why charging in the NHS has often been considered over the years, but rarely extended. A series of notes exchanged between Bevan and the Treasury in 1950 observed that if charges were more than nominal, there would have to be ways of exempting the least well-off. But these exemptions would bring 'administrative complexities and costs' and reduce the total yield.[18]

Derek Walker-Smith, a Conservative health minister in the late 1950s, argued for the abolition of charges: they were unpopular with medics and the public – a 'tax on illness'. They discouraged patients and doctors from taking necessary action; and they raised disappointing amounts of money.[19]

The same has been true in the pattern of the recovery of costs from insurance companies for treating patients involved in road traffic accidents. A review in 1982 concluded they would be wasteful of staff and management resources and that more than a fifth of the money raised would be spent on administration. These charges were nonetheless introduced under the 1988 Road Traffic Act, and have indeed raised only small amounts: around £20 million a year. This has not stopped the current Labour government urging trusts to work harder on collecting the fees and introducing centralised collection from the insurers.[20]

Attempts to introduce 'hotel charges' to cover the cost of accommodation in NHS hospitals have foundered on similar considerations. Such charges have been discussed throughout the history of the health service, most recently in 1993 when

Michael Portillo raised them as part of the Treasury's fundamental review of health spending. A fee of, say, £5 a day can
be justified on the grounds that the patient is saving money
on food and other spending while in hospital. And since it
would be incurred only after the GP recommended hospital
treatment, the charge would be less likely to deter people
from seeing a doctor. But if the exemptions are cast as widely
as for prescriptions, the amounts raised would be modest.
One estimate is that if the charge was set at £10 a day – a
level even many in work would find onerous – it would raise
no more than £200m.[21]

The health care people already pay for

Despite the resistance to charging in the NHS, people seem
prepared to spend quite large sums of their own money on
buying health care. These include over-the-counter medicines, holiday jabs, alternative therapies, family planning,
abortions and – most recently – walk-in doctor services.
These are in addition to the growth in conventional private
health care spending, whether it is made by paying direct or
through private health insurance.

The amount spent on over-the-counter medicines available without prescription reached £1,276 million in 1996.[22]
This is about a quarter of the NHS drugs bill and an average
of around £25 a year per person – more than £50 a year for
the average household. These proprietary medicines include
painkillers, skin creams and indigestion remedies and are
used to treat one in four ailments.

The list of medicines available over the counter has grown
in recent years, with more than 50 formerly available only on

prescription reclassified since 1983.[23] They include anti-histamines for hay fever and other allergies, nicotine gum and patches for those hoping to stop smoking and hydrocortisone preparations for skin complaints. Some quite sophisticated products are also available: acyclovir, the treatment for cold sores on sale as Zovirax cream; H2 antagonists for stomach ulcers such as Tagamet and Zantac; and imidazole antifungal treatments for vaginal thrush.

Many of these proprietary medicines are of limited value – few have been evaluated in formal clinical tests for use over the counter.[24] But while they may be no more than palliatives which relieve pain, fevers or runny noses, over-the-counter medicines are of value to users who wish to avoid disruption to their everyday life. For one thing, it is generally much more convenient to pop into the local chemist than to visit a GP (and the latter will usually require a visit to the former in any case, if the doctor writes a prescription). If patients want them and no harm is done in making them available, sale over the counter is simple and – in the current vogue language – empowers the consumer.

Pharmacists have actively lobbied for more drugs to be available over the counter in pharmacies, promoting the idea of the local chemist as part of the front-line health care team. Fears that they would abuse their role by always selling a medicine in response to a request seem unfounded. One study showed that no sale is made in a quarter of enquiries, and that chemists often recommend their customers visit their doctor.[25] GPs also seem increasingly open both to recommending patent medicines and to greater use of pharmacists by patients with minor ailments.[26]

Amounts spent on other forms of non-NHS treatment are harder to track down, and are concealed in the average of around £60 a year households spend on private medical, dental, nursing and optical fees.[27] Each year, for example, 70,000 people pay an average of £37.50 for holiday vaccinations at the British Airways network of 33 travel clinics. Many more pay their GP for the cost of the vaccine and perhaps also a small fee of around £7 for administration.

Some £500 million is spent every year on alternative therapies such as homeopathy and osteopathy, where patients typically spend up to £25 for a half-hour consultation. More than 50,000 women a year pay upwards of £300 (and sometimes much more) for an abortion through one of the charities or private hospitals – more than £15 million in total.

Finally, there is a fast-growing market for walk-in clinics. Sinclair Montrose Health care opened its first two Medicentres in London in 1997 at Victoria and Euston mainline stations offering a 15-minute consultation for £36. A longer consultation is £65, and the clinics offer full health checks for up to £250.

They have been so successful that more are to open in London and other large cities, with a total of 24 planned for the end of 1998. Bupa and PPP, the two biggest private health insurers, have their own plans along similar lines. It is, perhaps, revealing that the Sinclair Montrose clinics are advertised by a poster which shows a nurse telling a doctor: 'The patient is ready to see you now' – a reversal of the traditional NHS order of priorities.

Could we pay more?

The amounts most people pay privately are small beer in comparison with the cost of the NHS – more than £700 per person in the UK, or around £1,800 per household.[28] How easily could they pay more?

The MORI poll carried out for the Social Market Foundation in summer 1997 registered little support for further charging for health services. Four out of five opposed it in principle, with only one in eight supportive.[29] But just over half said they would be prepared to find the money if it improved the service – for example, by providing appointments outside working hours or to guarantee access to the most up-to-date treatments.[30] Perhaps as interesting, most thought there would be more charges introduced over the next 10 years.[31]

The simplest way to introduce new charges would be to ask people to pay to see a doctor. The figure of £5 for an appointment was tried out on the people in the Social Market Foundation poll, some of whom said they would be willing to pay it for visits outside office hours and others to guarantee same-day appointments. Seven out of ten said they would not be influenced by a fee of £5 for every non-emergency appointment – it would not affect how often they visited their GP.[32]

With the average person consulting a general practitioner five times a year,[33] a £5 fee for all appointments would cost the average household less than £50 a year. The British Medical Association – which does not support charging – calculated such a fee could raise £1.6 billion to help bridge the gap between resources and needs. A fee of £10 would raise

£3.3 billion, less if the charge led to fewer visits.

The SMF poll certainly indicated there would be fewer visits: a quarter of those asked about the £5 charge said they would come less often; half of those said *much* less often. Whether this would be the case remains to be seen – evidence discussed in the next chapter suggests the impact would be limited and could be mitigated by targeting special help.

Maintaining exemptions on similar grounds to those for prescription charges would reduce the disincentive effects for low income households. However, it could also enormously reduce the income – five out of six prescriptions are exempt from the charge. Having a period of the day when doctors could be seen free of charge on a no-appointment system might provide an alternative way of helping low-income patients. So, provided the exemption system was not overly generous, a £10 charge could raise around £2 billion a year.

Another way of raising extra cash would be to reduce the number of people who are exempt from prescription charges. Almost half of prescription items go to people over retirement age, for example. Around 44 per cent of pensioner households are on means-tested benefits, but a fifth have an above-average income.[34] If the exemption could be removed from better-off pensioners, charges might be paid on, say, double the current 16 per cent of prescribed items. This would raise another £421 million a year. Also lifting it for children other than those whose parents get means-tested benefits could double the amount raised.

It is difficult to know how much this would affect particular households. But since the average number of prescription items per pensioner household is 22 a year, most would be better off buying a £80.50 season ticket. This gives free prescriptions for a year and would cap the cost for those pensioners who had to pay.

A basic fee for using a hospital might also be considered, particularly for patients whose busy lifestyles make the idea of a firm appointment attractive. For example, £25 for day surgery and £50 for a longer stay would not penalise those with illnesses needing a long stay. On the assumption that those who could not afford such charges are not in work, they could be treated on a standby basis – no guaranteed appointment but no other penalty.

In 1994, 5.3 million people were admitted to NHS hospitals as in-patients, and 2.5 million treated as day-patients.[35] A rough calculation suggests charges at this level would have raised more than £300 million – perhaps half that after appropriate exemptions. Hospitals could also routinely offer patients enhanced facilities for a charge – just as when people are on holiday they may prefer to spend money on a better class of hotel or a taxi transfer.

Publishing price lists for the more common non-emergency operations – and suggesting that people think about private treatment – could find more patients willing to pay than at present. Already more than half the country's hip replacement operations are done privately. With private hospitals operating well below capacity, persuading more people to go private would free NHS beds for those who cannot pay.

Finally, people now pay 80 per cent of the cost of dental treatment on the NHS up to a limit of £330 per course. Once the other charges were established, a similar approach could be introduced for non-emergency surgery, with the idea of slowly raising the threshold to, say £500. This maximum could apply to any 12-month period to avoid bearing down too heavily on people needing several treatments.

Are such sums excessive? The average household already spends more than £700 a year on TV, video, hi-fi and other forms of entertainment.[36] An annual subscription to the full Sky satellite television package can cost over £500 a year – in addition to the £200-plus cost of the set-top box. More than 85 per cent of households with children have a video recorder – a figure that holds even for one-parent families. And football fans who buy season tickets for a premiership team spend on average £293 a year to attend 20 matches – around £15 a match.[37]

The average spent on tobacco by the 38 per cent of households that smoke is more than £800 a year. Even those households in the lowest tenth of the income range with a smoker spend more than £500 a year on tobacco. The average pet-owning household spends £300 a year on pet food and other such items – the bottom tenth spend around half that figure. When the pet is ill, owners pay fees of £20 or more to have treatment by a veterinarian – one reason why the waiting time to see a vet is usually shorter than to see a doctor.

When asked in the SMF poll about delays in operations for people experiencing minor discomfort, most said they would be happy to wait six months for treatment on the NHS. But 22 per cent said they would prefer to pay £500 for treatment within a month.[38] That, coincidentally, is the average amount spent by British households on their annual holiday – though the one in six that have a holiday abroad spend just under £2,500 a year.

An initial package of charges along the lines sketched out above could inject up to £5 billion a year into the NHS, adding 10 per cent to the budget. While it is fanciful to believe charging could turn patients into active consumers in emergency cases or complex surgery, most of these charges would be for services where the patient could exercise judgement over costs and quality without worrying about the medical implications. And it would be difficult to argue that asking for such payments – with appropriate exemptions for low-income households – would impose hardship in the closing years of the 20th century.

8: Paying for Services

The previous chapter proposed a range of additional charges for health care as a source of additional finance for the health service. The worry will inevitably be that these charges will deter some people from using the NHS and increase health inequalities. This chapter will look at the evidence from around the world on the impact of charges on health care. It will also examine what has happened in the UK since the mid-1980s following the steep increases in charges for NHS dentistry, eye tests and prescribed drugs.

The broad consensus in the medical profession is that charges are a disincentive to those needing access to care. A fair system for exempting low income groups can help those least able to pay, but it inevitably requires a complex bureaucratic machinery to run it. The collection and administration of charges thus swallows much of the proceeds in costs.[1]

There is particular concern about charging for basic screening services such as dental check ups and eye tests.[2] Screening plays an important role in improving the health of the population, and charges inevitably deter some from using such services. Opponents of charging argue this not only leads to worse health for those who are deterred, it may in the end be a false economy if the result is expensive treatment for conditions that could have been dealt with more cheaply if detected earlier. The academic view is summarised by Stephen Birch, one of the leading researchers on the impact of charges, as follows: 'There is considerable evidence that the imposition of user charges leads to significant reductions in service use and harmful effects on health status.'[3]

There is, indeed, plenty of evidence that charges affect people's use of medical services – it would be odd if they did not. Much of the evidence comes from overseas where studies have examined what happens when charges are introduced or removed.

One study of an experiment carried out by Stanford University in California concluded that an increase in the 'out-of-pocket price of care' resulted in a reduction in the demand for the forms of care affected.[4] Another in the Canadian province of Saskatchewan found the introduction of a charge of $1.50 for seeing a general practitioner led to a 14 per cent reduction in appointments among poor patients.[5]

The largest and most detailed study into the consequences of charges, carried out in the United States by the RAND Corporation, produced similar results. The California-based think-tank also found that people facing higher medical bills made less use of health care services – around a third fewer visits to a doctor and hospital stays.[6]

But while it is clear that charges reduce use of health services, it is not clear that these reductions lead to worse health among the population as a whole. The little evidence there is on the health consequences of charging comes largely from the RAND study, in particular from early reports on parts of the experiment that appeared to show that charges led to less healthy outcomes. However, the final conclusions of the study show a much more complex picture – and give little encouragement to those who want to oppose charges on health grounds.[7]

The evidence on charging

The RAND experiment can claim to be the only really scientific attempt to measure the impact of health care charges on the health of patients. RAND researchers wanted to investigate how much more medical treatment people might consume if charges decreased and whether this would improve their health overall. They set up a study which involved 2,000 non-elderly families from six areas chosen to be representative of the US.

Each of the families was given one of 14 health care plans which varied in the amount of money patients had to contribute towards treatment. At one end of the spectrum, all treatment was entirely free (something unusual in a US context); at the other end was a plan that required the patient to contribute 95 per cent of costs up to a yearly maximum of $1,000 per family (less for low-income families). In between were plans requiring lower contributions and with varying caps. The experiment, which was largely completed in the 1970s, covered the families for three or five years. It monitored the treatment they received and looked at the state of their health at the end of the experiment.

Perhaps it is not surprising that the more the families had to pay out of their own pocket, the fewer medical services they used. Families under the plan with the highest payments used between 25 and 30 per cent less services than those who had to contribute nothing. As payments rose, visits to the doctor, admissions to hospital, prescriptions and dental treatment fell. The main exception was for hospital admissions for children, which were unaffected by the level of contributions. Demand for mental health services was particularly vulnerable to charging, especially if payments were not capped – no doubt because people saw such treatment as likely to be long-term and an ongoing drain on their finances.

Much more surprising is the study's conclusions on the effects of varying levels of patient charges on health. For most people, using fewer health care services had 'little or no net adverse effect on health'.[8] Indeed, those who had to pay more reported fewer days of illness.

The results were sufficiently clear for the researchers to say there was no 'beneficial effect of free care on the General Health Index, our best summary measure of health'. Nor did those who paid more experience greater pain or worry – there was little or no variation according to the level of charges.

One small group did suffer adverse consequences from higher charges: what the study calls 'the sick poor'. Offering the most disadvantaged 6 per cent of the population free treatment substantially reduced their mortality rates. In particular, those who started the experiment with high blood pressure had it reduced more with free treatment than if they had had to make a contribution. There was a substantial improvement in death rates of 10 per cent for these people alone.

Free treatment also seemed to encourage better results for anaemic children in the most disadvantaged group. Charges had adverse effects on dental health – a decayed tooth was less likely to be filled and gum disease was marginally worse. A similar effect was found on ophthalmic health: free care improved near and far corrected vision in this group.

'For most individuals,' the study concluded, 'the cost of free care seems substantial and health benefits minimal.'[9] For those who might benefit – the sick poor – the recommendation was for a combination of targeted initiatives. These might include free screening for high blood pressure aimed at groups which were failing to have regular checks. Alternatively, there could be some exemptions from charges for low-income families or a lower cap on their charges.

US experience is, of course, no guide to the British NHS. And the consequences of introducing charges in a previously free health service might not be predictable from an experiment where charges are lifted in a system where they are routine. Nonetheless, the RAND experiment shows the intuitively obvious assumption – that higher charges damage health – is far from a full picture. For more than 15 out of 16 people, charging had no impact on their health.

For the small minority that suffered adverse effects from charges, the conclusion was that it was cheaper to target help on this group than to maintain the public expense of a free system for everyone. That is exactly what happens with the British system of charges for dentistry, eye care and prescription medicines – subject to large exemptions for the poor, the elderly and children. The rest of this chapter looks in more detail at these charges and the evidence on their impact on the health of the population.

Charges for dental care

Free dental treatment lasted for only the first three years of the National Health Service, before the introduction of charges for dentures in 1951. A flat-rate fee for dental treatment was added in 1952, but it was capped at relatively low levels until the 1980s. In April 1988, the charge rose to 75 per cent of the cost of treatment, with a maximum of £150 (including dentures). But in April 1989, the government abolished the free dental check up and the charge has since risen to 80 per cent of the cost with a maximum of £330.[10]

The following groups are exempt from the charges:

- children and young people under 19 in full-time education
- women who are either pregnant or have a child under 12 months
- people receiving Income Support, Family Credit, income-related Jobseeker's Allowance or Disability Working Allowance, and their partners
- families with a certificate for full help with the cost of NHS services.

A third of patients are covered by these exemptions. Despite the sharp rise in charges, they account for only about 20 per cent of the NHS spending on dentistry – down from 28 per cent in 1985 when charges were much lower.

The substantial increases in charges have been accompanied by growing dissatisfaction with NHS dentists, according to the British Social Attitudes survey. Satisfaction fell from 73 per cent in 1983 to 70 per cent in 1989 and 58 per cent in 1993.[11] However, it is not clear how much of this was caused by the dispute between dentists and the government over the fees they were allowed to charge for NHS treatment. Many dentists withdrew from the health service and went private to charge what they regarded as more reasonable fees. This made it increasingly difficult to find an NHS dentist in many parts of the country – particularly in London and the south-east where the highest levels of dissatisfaction were found.

The figures in Table 8.1 show what has happened since the charges were raised so steeply. The number of check-ups fell after charges were introduced in 1989, then rose and has since fallen back again. It is now 10 per cent below what it was in 1989. However, more than half of adults say they have a regular check-up – the highest level recorded.[12] Among children, the number registered with a dentist has risen by a quarter since the requirement to register was introduced in October 1990.

Table 8.1
NHS dental treatment in England

Year ending 31 March	Adult check-ups millions	Adult courses of treatment millions	Children registered millions
1989	20.9	24.0	–
1990	19.4	22.8	–
1991	19.0	22.6	–
1992	19.8	24.3	5.8
1993	20.0	25.1	7.1
1994	19.5	24.8	7.4
1995	19.3	24.9	7.4
1996	19.2	24.7	7.3
1997	18.9	24.6	7.3

Source: Department of Health, *1996 Health and Personal Social Services Statistics for England 1997*, London, The Stationery Office, 1998, Table B1.

The most convincing case against dental charges comes from a study carried out into the costs of NHS dental treatment before the steep rises of the late 1980s. This looked at the impact of the much more modest charges in force in 1985 on elderly patients – those over 65 – in England and Wales.[13] It found people who had to pay dental charges were four times more likely to receive occasional treatment than those who were exempt from paying. Occasional treatment is what dentists give when someone who is not a regular patient turns up with an immediate problem. The study concluded raising charges deterred patients from attending regular check-ups, increasing the need for such emergency attention.

The same study also found evidence that patients who had to pay received far less treatment than those who were exempt from charges – as Table 8.2 shows. Payers were 340 times more likely than non-payers to receive a check-up only, rather than more complex and expensive treatments. This raised the possibility that people who pay charges fail to follow up on necessary treatments because they find the cost prohibitive. Even when patients were given standard treatment, those exempt from charges received on average 60 per cent more treatment per course.

The study pointed out that these differentials could be explained by 'differences in the underlying health states of the two groups'. In other words, people who were exempt from charges may have had worse dental health than those who had to pay. Further, those who had to pay charges had an incentive to look after their teeth – unlike those who received treatment free.

Table 8.2

Dental treatment for patients 65 and over in England and Wales, 1985

Course type	Exempt patients (273,020) %	Non-exempt patients (1,823,500) %
Check-up only	0.07	23.80
X-ray, with or without check-up	0.40	0.44
Routine treatment	86.60	58.66
More elaborate treatment*	9.97	4.80
Occasional treatment	2.97	12.29

* Requiring prior approval.

Source: *Dental Estimates Board Annual Report, 1985*, cited in Birch, 1989, p. 137.

Another possible explanation of these results was that dentists – who are paid according to the number of services they give – had an incentive to treat non-paying patients no more than was necessary. They were less likely to over-treat patients they knew were paying for treatment personally. A third possibility was that dentists did not bother to submit details of all the treatment given to paying patients, since they could not reclaim the cost. This would mean the recorded figures for the cost of treatment for patients who were not exempt from charges were lower than the amount actually given.

The study concluded that such explanations could not account for all the variations between those who had to pay and those who were exempt. It was patient charges which were responsible, by deterring patients from going for check-ups.

However, this study provides no evidence that raising charges has led to worse dental health. Indeed, levels of dental health have improved greatly since the foundation of the National Health Service. The fall in dental decay is now beginning to 'bottom out', according to a recent House of Commons Health Select Committee report – but this is not unexpected given the improvement since 1948.[14] This observation is confirmed by the annual General Household Survey which, as Table 8.3 shows, has recorded a continuing decline in numbers of adults with no teeth of their own.

Table 8.3
The decline in adults with no teeth

Age	% in age group with no teeth					
	1983	1987	1989	1991	1993	1995
16–24	0	0	0	0	0	0
25–34	2	1	1	1	1	1
35–44	9	4	4	3	3	2
45–54	24	17	15	10	9	8
55–64	43	36	32	29	23	22
65–74	65	58	50	49	43	41
75 and over	82	78	75	67	67	64
All 16 and over	26	21	19	17	16	15

Source: Office for National Statistics, *Living in Britain 1995*, 1997, Table 9.1.

There remain large variations in dental health between different groups and regions. Table 8.4 shows that people in manual jobs are more than twice as likely to have no teeth as those in non-manual occupations. They are also less likely to have a regular check-up: 46 per cent of manual workers said they had one, against 61 per cent for people in non-manual jobs – the overall average was 54 per cent.[15]

Table 8.4
Total tooth loss by socio-economic group, Britain 1995

Socio-economic groups	% aged 16+ with no natural teeth
Professional	5
Employers and managers	8
Intermediate and junior non-manual	12
Skilled manual and own account non-professional	18
Semi-skilled manual and personal service	21
Unskilled manual	29
All non-manual	9
All manual	20
All aged 16 and over	15

Source: Office of National Statistics, *Living in Britain 1995: General Household Survey*, London, HMSO, 1997, Table 9.2.

Table 8.5 shows continuing variations between regions, with people in the north more than twice as likely to have no teeth as those in London and the south-east. To quote the then Chief Dental Officer, Mr Brian Mouatt: 'A rule of thumb might be that the further west or north you go the worse dental health tends to be.'[16] The number of adults with no teeth has fallen by more than 40 per cent since 1983 in the UK as a whole, slightly more in the south-east outside London, slightly less in the north. There is, overall, no sign that the north-south divide in dental health is closing.

Table 8.5
Total tooth loss by region

	British adults with no natural teeth %					
	1983	1987	1989	1991	1993	1995
Yorks. & Humberside	33	27	24	22	21	21
North	30	27	26	24	18	19
North West	30	22	23	21	19	17
West Midlands	27	21	18	18	15	15
East Midlands	27	22	20	19	17	14
East Anglia	25	19	18	14	13	13
South West	20	20	17	12	15	11
Greater London	17	14	14	12	11	10
Outer Metropolitan	17	13	13	12	9	10
Outer South East	21	18	14	12	13	10
England	24	20	18	16	15	14
Wales	30	28	23	21	19	18
Scotland	36	29	28	25	24	24
Great Britain	26	21	20	17	16	15

Source: Office for National Statistics, *Living in Britain 1995*, 1997, Table 9.11.

It seems unlikely that charges are to blame for these continuing inequalities, however. Bad dental health is highest among the lowest income groups. But those are also the groups which are most likely to be exempt from charges because they are on means-tested benefits.

As for regional inequalities with dental check-ups, Northerners are only slightly less likely on average to have a regular check-up. Londoners, who have the lowest rate of toothlessness, are the least likely to have a check-up – 41 per cent go regularly, while the average is 54 per cent.[17] The charges are identical in both regions, so cannot be the cause of the regional inequalities.

Charges also cannot explain the small rise in dental decay among children in certain areas identified by some witnesses to the Commons Health Committee in 1993.[18] Since children under 18 are exempt from charges, this suggests other factors are behind inequalities in their dental health.

The Commons Select Committee identified the following key factors as the cause of the inequalities in dental health: intake of fluoride via water and toothpaste; dietary habits; good oral health practice; the standard of dentists' work; and poverty. But if poverty is a factor, it is not because it makes it hard for people to pay the charges which exempt low-income groups. It must be because it affects the dietary habits and 'oral health practice' of individuals – a link between behaviour and ill-health that we will return to in the next chapter.

Overall, therefore, dental health has continued to improve since charges were hiked up, but there has been no reduction in inequality. These inequalities are a serious problem, but there is little evidence that rising charges have had much to do with them.

Charges for eye tests

Free eye tests, available to all, were part of the National Health Service from the start, along with free spectacles. Charges for glasses were introduced in 1951 together with those for dentures – ten shillings (50p) per lens plus the full cost of the frame apart from a limited range of NHS spectacles. Over the years, the charges crept up until in 1985 full charging was introduced for everyone apart from those on low incomes entitled to free NHS spectacles. In 1986, free spectacles were replaced with vouchers which could be used for a limited range of spectacles or put towards the cost of more expensive ones. And in 1989, the free eye test was abolished except for certain exempt groups.

The following are exempt from the charges:

- children under 16 and full-time students under 19
- people receiving Income Support, Family Credit, income-related Jobseeker's Allowance or Disability Working Allowance, and their partners
- registered blind and partially sighted people
- families on low income holding health benefits certificates
- glaucoma and diabetes sufferers and relatives aged over 40
- people requiring complex lenses.

Much less than half the population is exempt from paying for an eye test, and 3.8 million vouchers were redeemed in England in 1995–96.[19] Around two-thirds of people who are 16 or over wear glasses or contact lenses, rising to more than 95 per cent among over-65s.[20]

One aim of free eye tests was to encourage people from low-income groups to have their eyes checked regularly. They also provided a way of identifying preventable eye diseases such as glaucoma at an early stage.[21] Has the introduction of charges had adverse consequences for either of these aims?

Table 8.6
Number of eye tests

Year ending 31 March	millions
1988	13.5
1989	14.4
1990	10.8
1991	12.4
1992	12.8
1993	14.3
1994	13.2
1995	13.9
1996	14.6
1997	14.6

Source: Department of Health, cited in Harrison and New, 1997, p. 82.
Updated for 1997 by the DoH Sight Test Volume and Manpower Survey 1996–97.

There was certainly a dramatic drop in the number of eye tests after the charge was introduced, as Table 8.6 shows. Until 1989 the number of tests had been increasing by about 4 per cent a year, but it rose sharply in the year before the charge was introduced and then plummeted by a quarter in the following year. This was, as the British Medical Association and the Association of Optometrists put it: 'Undoubtedly due to the introduction of fees for private eye examinations'.[22]

The number of tests has since recovered and is now above 1989 levels. And the General Household Survey shows the proportion of the population who had had a sight test in the previous year rose from 27 per cent in 1990–91 to 32 per cent in 1993–94.[23]

Evidence gathered by NOP Consumer Market Research suggests people from lower-income groups are less likely to have their eyes tested: among the over-60s, 83 per cent in the professional and managerial social classes had been for an eye test, compared with 65 per cent in the semi-skilled and unskilled.[24] But since lower-income households have free tests, charging is unlikely to have been a significant cause of this.

As for the impact on health, a study at the Bristol Eye Hospital found the introduction of the eye test fee had led to a drop in referrals for serious eye problems – numbers were between 13.7 per cent and 19 per cent fewer than expected on past trends.

Perhaps more serious was a similar decline in referrals for glaucoma, the potentially blinding disease which can be prevented fairly simply and cheaply if caught in its early stages. Cases identified for further attention declined by nearly a fifth after the introduction of the fee, leading the researchers to conclude that 'an increased prevalence of preventable blindness may result'.[25]

Glaucoma affects around 2 per cent of those aged over 40,

more than half of whom have a type which the patient usually notices only when there has been appreciable and irreversible loss of vision. Eye testing can detect the disease long before this stage, but about half of the cases remain undiagnosed, according to Professor Richard Wormald, Director of the Glaxo Department of Ophthalmic Epidemiology at Moorfields Eye Hospital. There is concern that the charge for sight testing is deterring those most at risk – the over-65s, people of African origin and lower socio-economic groups.

However, the failure to detect around half the cases of glaucoma appears to be a common experience elsewhere. A survey of nine studies in the United States and Europe between 1966 and 1994 found that close to or more than half of patients with glaucoma had been previously undetected – irrespective of whether there were charges for eye tests.[26] This is partly due to inadequate screening for the disease – examiners who test comprehensively detect about 50 per cent more cases than average. It is also caused by the reluctance of optometrists to refer many patients who are in apparently low-risk categories to overloaded hospital eye clinics.

Professor Wormald rejects any simple nationwide screening strategy to tackle the problem. His recommendations include free eye tests for elderly people, initiatives in areas with high proportions of Afro-Caribbean people and campaigns to raise awareness.[27] Such a targeted approach looks much more likely to reduce cases of glaucoma than free eye tests for everyone which rarely reach more than half the population and have had little impact on detection levels of glaucoma.

Prescription charges

The ability to levy a charge for prescriptions was introduced in 1949 by Nye Bevan, who nonetheless managed to persuade the Treasury that there was no need to impose one. Shortly after Labour left power in 1951, the new Conservative government used the legislation to bring in a one shilling (5p) charge per prescription. And apart from the years 1965–68, there have been charges ever since – with a large group of people exempt from paying the charges since their reintroduction in 1968.

The charge has risen steeply since 1979, from 45p an item to £5.65 in April 1997 – a 250 per cent increase in real terms. This covers about half the cost of the average prescription item which is around £9.30. But the charge is almost double the cost of the average generic – that is unbranded – item which costs £2.96, which means that some patients pay more for drugs on prescription than they might over the counter.

Despite this, prescription charges raise just 8 per cent of the annual NHS pharmaceuticals bill – £310 million in 1996–97.[28] The reason is that five out of six prescriptions are exempt from charges because they are for a patient in one of the following categories:

- children under 16 and those under 19 in full-time education
- women who are either pregnant or have a child under 12 months
- men and women aged 60 and over
- people receiving Income Support, Family Credit, income-related Jobseeker's Allowance or Disability

Working Allowance, and their partners
- anyone exempt from NHS charges on low-income grounds
- war pensioners – exempt for medication for a war disability
- people with certain medical conditions, including forms of diabetes, epilepsy and physical disabilities that confine the patient to home
- people with a prepayment certificate which gives free prescriptions for a year on payment of £80.50 for the 1997–98 year.

Of the 560 million items prescribed in 1996, almost half go to the over-60s. In 1979, elderly people received an average of 12½ items each; this had increased to 22 by 1996. Young people exempt from the charge account for around 12 per cent of items.[29]

The cost of NHS drugs has drifted upwards over the years, as Table 8.7 on the following page shows – a pattern seen in most advanced countries' health services. This is partly owing to a doubling in the number of prescription items since the foundation of the NHS, and partly to the increasing cost of drugs, with the average cost per item having risen by 50 per cent in real terms since 1975. The result is that the real cost per capita of NHS prescriptions has almost doubled over that period.

Each rise in the prescription charge is greeted with cries of anger from doctors, pharmacists and patient groups. The British Medical Association has called for a fundamental review of the whole system of charging, which it argues is unfair and anomalous. For example, the exemptions do not cover important groups with chronic conditions such as

Table 8.7
Cost of NHS prescriptions

Year	Number of prescriptions per head	Cost per head £	% of total NHS bill
1949	4.5	0.27	8.0
1959	4.7	1.62	10.2
1969	5.5	3.43	10.6
1979	6.7	16.34	9.9
1989	7.6	47.66	10.7
1992	8.4	64.29	10.5
1996	9.5	86.69	12.1

Source: Office of Health Economics, *Compendium of Health Statistics*, 1997, Tables 4.26, 4.29.

cystic fibrosis and Parkinson's disease. Yet other groups are exempt despite being able to afford to pay (as many pensioners are) or not at particular risk (women during pregnancy and for the year after the birth). As noted above, the charge is often more than the cost of the items prescribed.

The BMA is concerned that the rises dissuade patients from visiting the doctor when they are ill. 'All GPs have anecdotal evidence of patients asking which two or more items on a prescription form are the most important as they cannot afford to pay for more than one at a time,' it says.[30]

There are, in fact, several studies on the impact of increases in the prescription charge on the consumption of prescribed drugs. One using data between 1971 and 1982 found a 10 per cent increase in the prescription price reduced the number of paid-for prescriptions by between 1.5 and 2 per cent.[31] A more comprehensive study covering 1969 to 1986 appeared to confirm such figures.[32] It found a 10 per cent rise in the charge reduced the number of non-exempt prescriptions by 2.3 per cent between 1969 and 1977, and by 6.4 per cent between 1978 and 1986. The author suggested this higher rate during the second half of the study reflected the much higher annual increases in the charge which began under the 1979 Conservative government – leading more people to decide not to pay the charge.

The study also showed that a rise in the prescription charge led to an increase in sales of over-the-counter patent medicines. Overall between 1969 and 1986, a 10 per cent increase in the charge led to a 3.3 per cent fall in demand for paid-for prescription items, but a 2.2 per cent increase in over-the-counter medicines. This could be because GPs suggest buying a cheaper patent medicine rather than giving a prescription, or patients themselves decide to buy a cheaper over-the-counter product.

A third study covered adult, non-elderly patients in England between 1979 and 1985, a period when the prescription charge was raised 490 per cent in real terms.[33] The number of prescriptions per head among those not exempt from the charge fell by a third over those six years. Nonetheless, this study produced a much lower figure for the impact of raising the charge – it found a 10 per cent rise reduced paid-for prescriptions by 1 per cent.

A more recent study of data between 1969 and 1992 saw a higher figure of a 3.2 per cent fall in paid-for prescriptions following a 10 per cent increase in the charge.[34] Thus the 1992 increase in the charge from £3.75 to £4.25 brought in £17.3 million of extra revenue and cut the 55 million prescriptions not exempt from the charge by 2.3 million. The authors, David Hughes and Alistair McGuire, suggest that if some of those deterred from using prescription drugs ended up being treated for more serious conditions in hospital, the cost of that treatment could erode the savings.

Whatever the level of the effect, it must surely be the case that prescription charges do reduce the rate of usage of prescribed drugs among non-exempt patients. The sharp decline in the proportion of prescriptions which are non-exempt suggests as much. Since 1979, the number of prescriptions incurring the charge has more than halved in England from 109 million to less than 50 million, while the number of prescriptions overall has risen around 40 per cent. Barely 11 per cent of prescriptions are now paid for, compared with almost half in 1969.[35]

The question is whether this matters – do people who really need drugs not get them as a result of prescription charges? The study which found a rise in sales of over-the-counter drugs as the prescription charge rose suggests much of the fall in prescribed drugs is accounted for by a switch to patent medicines. It is, of course, impossible to say that these patent medicines were the same as what might have been prescribed – or as effective. But apart from the anecdotes referred to by the BMA in its call for a rethink on prescription charges, there is no evidence that the fall in prescribed items has had adverse effects on the health of the nation. As one of the researchers summarises it: 'UK evidence on, and research into, the health effects of user charges is sadly lacking.'[36]

The case against charges

Thus in all three of the areas where charging is routine in the National Health Service, the consequence has been to reduce usage – in the short term, at least. But there is little evidence that the charges have adversely affected the health of those that pay them – indeed, the worst health afflicts those who are most likely to be exempt from the charges. Dental health has continued to improve while the number of people having eye tests is now higher than pre-charging levels, with an increasing range of low-cost services and products.

This does not deter those who advocate an end to the charging. Stephen Birch argues – referring to charges for dental care and prescriptions – that increases in patient charges by Conservative governments in the 1980s had created a 'two-tier system of finance of primary health care', that will inevitably deter uptake of the services affected:

> The individual consults the doctor [however] only
> where the expected benefits of consulting, in terms of
> perceived improvements in health status offered by the
> doctor's advice or prescription, exceed the costs incurred
> by the individual in consulting the doctor and following
> his advice.[37]

Elsewhere, he argues that among elderly people, the imposition of dental charges 'distorts the cost to the user of these services relative to other goods and hence creates additional barriers or disincentives to use.'[38]

A more interesting way of looking at it might be to say that failing to impose charges distorts choice. As noted earlier, there is considerable waste in a free service, highlighted by the 'frequent attender' phenomenon. Between 6 per cent and 20 per cent of patients fail to redeem prescriptions and up to half delay or omit doses.[39]

The final report of the RAND experiment suggests that there may even be beneficial effects from charges if they reduce the amount of 'inappropriate care'. This produces no benefit for patients and may even put them at risk – hence the higher number of days off sick when charges are reduced. The authors highlight evidence which suggests that 4 per cent of people admitted to hospital have their illness prolonged by injuries incurred during treatment. Another study calculated that the benefits produced by many medical procedures are not enough to justify the risk involved in using them.[40]

The experience of European countries where charges are commonplace suggests they do not create a two-tier service. As already observed, health inequality is less in most of those countries than in Britain's free-of-charge National Health Service.[41]

9: Closing the Health Gap

Previous chapters have suggested that individuals should be encouraged to make a larger contribution to their health care. The greatest fear for most people will be that this will lead to a less fair health service, where those with least money will receive inferior treatment. Would extra charges fatally undermine equality in the NHS?

Superficially, the answer appears clear-cut: if people have to pay, there will be greater inequality, because some can afford to pay more than others. We have already seen, however, that paying does not necessarily lead to greater inequality. Most other European health services require payments, with better or no worse outcomes in terms of equality.

The additional resources provided by charging could increase the amount of treatment available. This does not inevitably mean more health care for the wealthier in society: the extra treatment could allow health care services to be spread more widely. And if usage of particular medical services falls, the reason may be a reduction in unnecessary use rather than inability to pay for necessary health care.[1]

The RAND study described in Chapter 8 appears to support this thesis: there was no impact on the health of most people when charges were higher, even though they led to less trips to the doctor and fewer stays in hospital. There were, however, damaging effects for a small minority of the 'sick poor' – around 6 per cent of the sample. But these people could be protected by measures which targeted those who might suffer from charges.

Ensuring that the benefits of charging are spread widely – and that low-income groups do not lose out – will be the continuing role of government. Now, as in 1948, health care

cannot be left to the market to provide, because it has characteristics that distinguish it from other goods and services –
even essentials such as food, water and shelter. These are the
unpredictability of health care, the reliance of patients on the
doctor for guidance and the fundamental importance of
health services which means people cannot be allowed to go
without them.

This chapter examines each of these characteristics in
order to throw light on the role of government in providing
health care. It will also look at the factors behind existing inequalities to see whether charging will make them worse or
better.[2]

The unpredictability of health care

The inherent unpredictability of ill-health is the first reason
why health care cannot be left to the market. We know much
of the demand for health services is likely to fall in the final
years of a patient's life, but the quantity can vary tremen-
dously between individuals. Much more unpredictable are
accidents and other afflictions and illnesses needing treatment that few could hope to pay for out of their own
pocket.

When the risks faced by individuals are unpredictable, insurance offers a solution. Provided the overall risk to the
group is quantifiable, it can be pooled as it is with car accidents or household subsidence, so that policyholders pay into
a fund which those who run into trouble can draw on. There
are problems, however, in health insurance which mean it
can rarely be left to voluntary private insurance.

One difficulty is that insurers can pool risks only when

the overall risk to the group is predictable. But with health, there is always a danger of an unforeseen epidemic or condition such as AIDS. Traditional insurance deals with national or regional catastrophes such as typhoons or earthquakes through reinsurance which spreads the risk between insurers all over the globe. But a global epidemic could not be dealt with in this way.

Another difficulty is that certain individuals are uninsurable because they have congenital defects or are chronically ill. A third is moral hazard: if someone else is paying for medical treatment, there is no incentive to adopt a healthy lifestyle – or to cut the cost of treatment.

All of these drawbacks are shared by state-backed national insurance schemes and tax-funded health services. But the difference with private insurance is that it is voluntary, and people can act in ways that undermine the pooling of risk. Some people are healthier than others, and will not want to share the cost of supporting those who make more claims. And insurers will aim to select the healthiest individuals to keep down their claims. The result of this 'adverse selection', as it is known, is that it creates a group of poor-risk people who cannot get insurance at a reasonable cost – or even get it at all.

These are the reasons why governments step in to ensure everyone is covered against the unpredictability of health care needs. The most important measure to achieve this is compulsory membership of health insurance schemes – which only the state can enforce. In much of Europe, this is done through social insurance where everyone pays into one or more common funds which cover entire nations or classes of people.

In some cases the payments are special health or social security contributions; in others such as the UK, the payment is through general taxation. If there is more than one insurance fund there may need to be government action to share risk between them.[3] In the Netherlands where there are competing sickness funds, for example, the government covers what it calls catastrophic risks through a compulsory state-regulated system funded by taxation.[4]

In countries where private insurers operate, the government is forced to be the insurer of last resort for those who cannot afford it. In Switzerland, for example, the government subsidises the premiums of low income groups. In the US, two federal schemes are funded by the taxpayer: Medicare for the elderly and Medicaid for the poor. Those who cannot get insurance are usually the greatest health risks, so the cost of this safety-net insurance is high. The American government thus ends up spending a higher proportion of GDP on publicly funded health care than the UK. Since this is financed from taxes which are mainly collected from people covered by private insurance, these people end up paying twice.

Other countries which have adopted private-insurance based systems have had similar results.[5] Chile, for example, has a classic two-tier system in which high-income workers enjoy good-quality services offered by private insurers while the rest are left in a lower quality public plan. And in the Philippines, the health maintenance organisations which both pay for and provide health care have excluded the elderly.

There is one further consequence of a competitive insurance system: proliferation in administration and marketing costs. These typically account for less than 10 per cent in state-financed systems but in Chile and the Philippines, administrative and sales costs eat up 20 per cent or more of premiums.[6]

The imbalance of information

The second reason why health care is different is the 'information asymmetry' identified in Chapter 7 as an obstacle to charging for health services. Classical economic theory assumes the individual is the best judge of what is in his or her best interest. But this is not always true in health services where patients often know little about what is wrong with them or what the cure should be. This makes it hard to establish the normal buying and selling relationship of a commercial transaction.

Even if patients knew more about medicine, the nature of their illness or condition could make it hard for them to act like consumers and shop around when they need medical treatment.[7] This is especially true for those who are mentally ill, handicapped, disabled or facing a life-threatening illness. It is also true for those in the final years of their lives in which so much medical treatment is concentrated, when they may be vulnerable by virtue of their age and frailty. But it applies just as much to the patient in the prime of life who wants only to be restored to health – not to engage in economic exchange.

Thus patients must rely on the medical profession to make choices for them. And because it is either an insurance company, social insurance fund or the taxpayer who pays the bill, the doctor has no incentive to minimise costs. Indeed, experience shows that letting patients have all the health care they want leads in practice to the enrichment of the medical profession. Countries such as Singapore and Korea which have tried to let market forces rule in health services have found costs rocketing as physicians' incomes rise much faster than the average.[8]

The extent to which health care is supply-led rather than driven by patient demand is reflected in the findings from many countries that the more doctors there are, the more health care is provided. Once there are doctors, they will find health care services to offer and patients will take them up even when they have to pay. If one form of treatment is shown not to work or is no longer needed, the medics simply start providing other types of health care – just as dentists have moved into cleaning and cosmetic work on teeth as better dental health has led to fewer fillings.

Information asymmetry is not unique to health services, of course – it is found in other commercial sectors. Consumers routinely buy complex electronic products and ever-more sophisticated cars with little grasp of how they work or what makes one better than another. We rely on manufacturers and retailers to supply us with safe and nutritious foodstuffs (not always with justification), and most people have only a scant understanding of the complex financial products they buy – from insurance policies to pension plans.

In these cases, however, there are alternative sources of information to help consumers make their choices. Magazines such as *Which?*, *Autocar* and *What Computer?* test products, compare data and offer advice on what to buy. Retailers and other intermediaries act as agents for their customers, buying the best brands and giving advice at the time of purchase. The state regulates in the public interest to ensure minimum standards and redress the imbalance of power between the individual consumer and the powerful corporation. And when the information asymmetry is exploited as badly as it was over the mis-selling of pensions, the government intervenes to force pension providers to put matters right.

In health services, more information is becoming available to patients through periodicals, books and the internet. The parents of the five-day-old baby who was given a liver transplant in December 1997 found a surgeon willing to perform the operation by surfing the net. The government can try to influence medical practice through regulation of doctors, initiatives to cut down on ineffective procedures and by rationing decisions. And the concept behind GP fundholding was that the family doctor would act as the intermediary for patients – shopping around on their behalf and making sure they weren't mis-sold treatment.

In the end, however, medical practice is not a commercial transaction but a relationship between an individual patient and the physician deploying all the skills of the profession. While the long-term consequences of a bad pension choice can be very damaging to the individual affected, a wrong decision over whether or not to follow a particular course of treatment may be fatal. This is what Professor Julian Le Grand of the LSE describes as the 'fundamental importance' of health care.

The unhealthy are different

The idea that health care is fundamentally important in a way that is different even to that of other necessities of life is deeply rooted in human society. It is why most people believe inability to pay should not be a reason to deny medical treatment. And it contributes to the difficulty in changing health services, since anyone who loses out from change weighs much more heavily in public debate than the potential gainers who may be in much greater number.

The fundamental importance of health is that it is a precondition for other activities – for leading a life as unhampered by illness or disability as possible. Ill-health is not a choice for which individuals can always be held responsible, even if they have contributed by smoking, being overweight or taking intravenous drugs, for example. Individuals may indulge in behaviour which has serious effects on their health, but few people would argue the patient should be left to stew. Health is different and we should not be allowed to suffer the consequences of eventualities beyond our control – or even eventualities we might have controlled but failed to.

It is the combination of this fundamental importance of health care with the unpredictability of ill-health and the information asymmetry of health services which forces governments to intervene. They do not routinely over-ride market forces when individuals fail to act in their own best interests in buying food, drink, shelter or heat. Food is as fundamentally important to human life as health, but the need is predictable and there is little information imbalance. As Bill New and Julian Le Grand point out, this is why there is no National Food Service.[9]

There are other activities which are unpredictable and where the consumer is at an information disadvantage – in the repair of cars after an accident for example. Accidents are by definition unpredictable, and we have already noted that most of us know little about the workings of our cars. It is equally well-known that the car repair market is not a perfect one – as soon as the repairer learns the vehicle is insured, the bill goes up and the standard of repair is more than an individual car-owner would pay for. But there is no need for state intervention in because the activity is not of such fundamental importance to justify it.

This suggests a framework for deciding what it should be the state's responsibility to provide in health care – the core NHS that people cannot be reasonably expected to provide for themselves. Public funding is appropriate for all forms of treatment that meet the three criteria; other services can be left to the individual.

Thus, for example, long-term residential care for the elderly does not fit into the framework, fundamentally important though it is to the individual. The likelihood of needing it is entirely predictable, and most people have a pretty clear understanding of what they want from such care. There may be a role for the state in helping those who are confused or handicapped and cannot make choices for themselves. And people might have to be compelled – or at least heavily persuaded – to make sufficient provision, given the difficulty many younger people have in saving for far-distant eventualities. But there is no compelling reason for governments to interfere in a service which people can quite easily provide for themselves.

Emergency treatment, expensive operations and therapies that save or extend lives and treatment after accidents all fall into the framework. They are not predictable, they are of fundamental importance and the information imbalance is acute.

The principles would not, however, extend to cosmetic surgery or dentistry merely for enhancement purposes – again the individual is not only able to judge its value but is also the person best-placed to do so. Nor would they extend to fertility treatments such as *in vitro* fertilisation which cannot be argued as being of such fundamental importance to the life of the putative parent, important though child-bearing might be psychologically.

The provision of dentures, hearing aids and spectacles is also a service which can be left to individuals. They are fundamentally important appliances, but the customer can buy them with confidence. The same is true of palliative medicines such as painkillers and skin creams.

There is, however, a good case for saying that check-ups – eye tests, regular dental checks and even visits to the GP – qualify under the three criteria. Each of them may detect conditions the patient is unaware of, and must rely on the opinion of the doctor, dentist or optician. The same is true of prescribed drugs, where the patient should not be encouraged to substitute his or her opinion for that of the physician.

Does this mean that to charge for these – and also for cheap forms of dental and medical treatment – should be ruled out because they meet the three criteria? It would be absurd, particularly as we have already found no convincing evidence that the relatively modest charges for these medical services have had any adverse effect on health. One further criterion is needed: the state should pay for health care only when individuals cannot be expected to pay for it themselves.

In a society as wealthy as the UK, there is a good case for leaving out of the core package relatively cheap forms of treatment. People who routinely spend £15 for a ticket to a football match or £6 to hire a couple of videos for the weekend can easily afford health care charges of comparable size. Apart from anything else, the cost of reimbursing such modest charges in a free health service is disproportionate. And with the NHS budget under pressure, raising such charges could be the way to bridge the funding gap and ensure that much more expensive and important forms of treatment are more readily available.

Making life worse for the poor?

The benefits of having the extra income from charging look very attractive. But will such an approach not increase the existing inequalities in health – which we have already seen are greater in the UK than in other parts of Europe? If charging is to be politically acceptable, supporters must demonstrate that it will not increase health inequality.

The starting point for analysing the impact of charges must be an examination of the causes of health inequalities.[10] The dominant view in public health circles is that they are caused by social inequality. This view is reflected in the government's recent green paper which starts from the assertion that an individual's health is 'basically influenced by how well off they are, where they live and by their ethnic background'.[11] It produces evidence to show that:

Poor people are ill more often and die sooner. The life expectancy of those higher up the social scale (in professional and managerial jobs) has improved more than those lower down (in manual and unskilled jobs). This inequality has widened since the early 1980s.[12]

The green paper also produces figures showing inequalities between ethnic groups. And evidence of a growing polarisation between different areas of the country has been collated in a recent study funded by the Joseph Rowntree Foundation.[13] This showed that by the early 1990s, people under 65 living in the areas with the highest premature death rates were 42 per cent more likely to die than the UK average. In the early 1950s, the figure was 31 per cent.

As Table 9.1 shows, the gap between the best and the worst areas has widened over the last 40 years. One in twelve of the population now lives in an area where deaths are more than 15 per cent above expected levels – the highest number since the 1950s. And the worst health areas are those where households are least likely to own a car, most likely to be unemployed with children and most likely to have an adult with a long-term illness.

Certainly a clear connection can be established between poverty and some forms of ill-health – a fact we are frequently reminded of by television pictures from around the world. Poverty forces people into damp and unsanitary housing in polluted surroundings, to drink dirty water and rely on an inadequate diet. These conditions cause illnesses such as cholera and typhoid which often lead to premature death.

Table 9.1
Health inequalities and poverty

Decile	Standardised mortality ratio* for deaths under 65		Poverty indicators, %		
			Residents in households with no	Children in households with no	Adults under 65 with a long-term
	1950–53	*1990–92*	*car*	*work*	*illness*
Bottom tenth	131	142	41	33	9.7
2	118	121	31	24	8.4
3	112	111	31	21	8.0
4	107	105	26	20	8.3
5	103	99	23	19	6.9
6	99	94	22	16	6.4
7	93	91	20	16	6.0
8	89	86	17	12	5.6
9	86	80	13	10	4.9
Top tenth	82	76	11	8	4.5
Average	100	100	24	17	6.9

* This table divides the population into ten equal-sized groups known as deciles. The bottom group is made up of the worst tenth of areas in terms of the death rates per 1,000 people under 65, while the top decile is the best tenth. The standardised mortality ratio shows the death rates adjusted to allow for the differing sex and age of the areas and then expressed as a percentage of the average for the whole country.
Source: Daniel Dorling, *Death in Britain: How Local Mortality Rates have Changed 1950s-1990s*, 1997, Tables 14, 16.

There has been much excitement in the last half century over advances in surgery and new drugs such as antibiotics. But the greatest increases in life expectancy have followed public health measures such as cleaner water, better housing, improved sanitation and reductions in environmental pollution. As societies become wealthy enough to afford these basic standards, the health of their peoples is hugely improved.

There remain pockets of acute deprivation even in wealthy societies such as the UK, where low incomes, bad diet and substandard housing produce diseases such as tuberculosis thought to have been eradicated decades ago. While infant mortality rates are so low in the UK that there is no significant variation between regions, there are areas within regions where high rates could be reduced by appropriate measures. There are also the particular problems for low-income groups living in 1960s system-built housing which is as damp as the worst Victorian tenements.

But most people in Britain face a different set of health challenges. The infectious diseases that used to carry off the poor at a young age have been largely conquered. Premature death is now most common in late middle-age, mostly as a consequence of degenerative illnesses such as cancer and heart disease. However, the links between these diseases and income is less clear.

Some of the degenerative illnesses afflict the less affluent more seriously. Unskilled people are twice as likely as the average to die from lung cancer, for example, and 80 per cent more likely to die from heart disease. The gap is much lower for social class four – the semi-skilled – but still clear; 32 per cent more likely to die of lung cancer and 21 per cent more with heart disease.[14]

With other illnesses, the relationship is the other way round. For example, professionals, managers and skilled people are more likely to die from skin cancer than the semi-skilled and unskilled.[15] And the highest rates of deaths from breast cancer among women aged 55-64 are in the more affluent groups. This has been a consistent finding in comparisons between European countries and between regions or social classes within countries such as Britain.[16]

Nor is the social incidence of particular diseases fixed. Heart disease now hits lower income groups hardest, but it used to be associated with higher incomes. In the 1950s, death rates from this cause were higher in classes one and two – professionals and managers – than in classes four and five – the semi-skilled and unskilled. Forty years on, heart disease is more likely to attack the less affluent members of society.

The same has happened with premature death from lung cancer for men between 55 and 64, which now also bears down more heavily on lower income groups in the UK. International evidence again shows it to be an affliction of wealth. In the 1950s, death rates from lung cancer in the more affluent countries of northern Europe such as Finland, Austria and England was double that of the poorer southern countries such as Italy, Spain and Greece. Since then, rising standards of living in the southern countries has raised the rates and there is now little variation between the two regions.[17]

Even where there is a correlation between income and a

particular disease, the exact cause and effect may be unclear. With coronary heart disease, for example, the death rate has steadily declined since the 1970s in all regions of the UK. If there was a direct link with lower incomes, this trend would have been interrupted by the recessions of the early 1980s and early 1990s or the increase in unemployment in each successive downturn.

If there is no direct link between income and an illness such as heart disease, perhaps the cause is relative deprivation, the widening gap between rich and poor that began to open during the 1980s. While households on the lowest incomes are consuming more than they did 20 years ago in absolute terms, they have received less of the fruits of society than the better-off – with adverse effects on their health. The government's green paper refers to this as social exclusion, when those at the bottom of the income ladder are excluded from the opportunities open to those further up.

But income differentials are not enough to explain the variations in health between the classes. There are big differences between the death-rates of semi-skilled workers and the unskilled, but these two groups are quite close together in terms of gross weekly income. In contrast, there is a much larger gap between the income of the top two classes – professionals and managers – but their death-rates are much closer.

Could it be that a small increase in income has the largest impact on death-rates for those with the lowest incomes? In this case, those on higher incomes would need a much greater increase to produce much of an impact on death-rates. But if this explanation was correct, we would expect rising incomes over the years to reduce the gap between the classes on death-rates. This has not happened: the difference between the death rates of professionals and unskilled workers stayed the same between 1951 and 1971 – even though real earnings rose by 50 per cent.[18] There was a similar result in Sweden, where the differences between classes regarding their death-rates rose slightly from the late 1960s to the late 1970s.

Men and women behaving badly

The higher incidence of heart disease and lung cancer among the unskilled and semi-skilled cannot simply be explained by their income. It can, however, be explained by their behaviour: people in classes four and five are now more likely to smoke and be overweight, for example, than those in classes one and two. While 29 per cent of men smoke, the figure is 46 per cent for the unskilled and 36 per cent for semi-skilled. Just 12 per cent of professionals and 22 per cent of managers smoke – and they smoke fewer cigarettes than the average smoker.[19]

Many of the degenerative diseases responsible for premature death are linked to behaviour such as smoking, excessive drinking, over-eating and lack of exercise. These patterns of consumption reflect affluence rather than poverty. The diseases they are associated with thus become more prevalent as societies become richer.

Once these forms of behaviour are identified as causes of ill-health, however, they tend to decline in wealthier countries. This is what happened with smoking in northern Europe, and it was followed by a fall in lung cancer rates. But within particular societies, those in lower social classes are less likely to abandon the unhealthy forms of behaviour. They thus become more prone to the degenerative diseases and health inequality rises as a result.

That means health policy cannot rely on a simple model which relates inequality in health to inequality in income. With some diseases such as cholera or typhoid, there is a direct connection between poverty and illness. This can be broken by changing the conditions the poor are forced to live under. With other diseases such as coronary heart disease and lung cancer, there is a correlation between premature death and social class or income but no direct causal connection. The link can be broken only by changing the behaviour of those who are prone to the illness which contributes to its incidence.

Establishing that it is behaviour rather than income that is behind health inequality is, however, little help in thinking about the future of the health service. If certain forms of behaviour are associated with low incomes and they cause ill-health, introducing charges could still make things worse. The question is, then, whether there are better ways to reduce health inequality than offering free health care.

One fact that needs to be remembered is that despite the apparent growth in health inequality, people's health is, in general, improving. The study which showed a widening gap between the best and worst areas of the UK also shows that all areas have seen immense improvements in life chances over the last 40 years. Those in the worst tenth of areas now have less chance of dying under the age of 65 than those in the best tenth had in the early 1950s. Everyone's life chances have improved by at least 80 per cent since the 1950s – but the improvement has been greatest in more affluent areas.[20]

There is also evidence that the real problem of health inequality is faced by a declining number of people. If the worst two areas – deciles one and two – are left out, all the others have improved their performance in relation to the average since 1950–53. The top 60 per cent are less likely than average to die under 65 in 1990–92. In 1950–53, it was only the top 50 per cent which were less likely to die than average. There has been a growth in inequality between the top and bottom of the scale, but everyone apart from those at the bottom has improved their chances.

Many of those people at the bottom of the scale will be the unskilled who form social class five. Here again, the gap is not quite as it seems: class five has changed enormously since the foundation of the NHS.[21] In 1951, for example, a quarter of men aged 55 and over fell into it – reflecting the enormous number of unskilled jobs in heavy industry during their working lives. Even among younger men, more than 10 per cent were in class five, a substantial group of people with a place in society and full-time paid work.

Today less than one in twenty of the population counts as unskilled, and the social condition of people in class five has changed enormously. To be unskilled now is to be at the very bottom of the pile in the world of work, part of the new underclass which has no security of employment and is thus excluded from society. Comparing the health of the substantial group in class five 50 years ago with that much smaller underclass today is to compare apples and pears.

Any apparent widening of the health gap between classes

four and five and the rest of society should therefore be balanced by a recognition that the numbers so disadvantaged are shrinking. And the fact that so many people at the bottom of the social scale suffer poor health – often related to unhealthy forms of behaviour – raises the question of cause and effect. The Labour government unambiguously identifies poverty as the cause of ill-health in its January 1998 green paper: 'It's harder to stop smoking when you're worrying about making ends meet.'[22]

This argument seems bizarre: what is it about smoking which makes it more attractive when ends become hard to meet given the cost of cigarettes after successive hikes in tobacco taxation? If there is a correlation between low incomes and behaviour such as smoking, it is implausible that it is the former that causes the latter. At the same time, it is no more plausible that unhealthy behaviour causes low incomes, unless it reaches the point of making an individual unemployable.

This suggests there is a third factor which leads individuals to end up on low incomes and also produces the unhealthy behaviour which is the factor behind ill-health. One candidate is educational achievement. The correlation between education and income is well-established though not overwhelming. In other words, getting a good education helps in earning a good income – but it doesn't guarantee it. A good education is more likely to produce good health, however, when health, income and education are analysed together. Indeed some studies have found higher income produces worse health if years of schooling are taken into account.[23]

This suggests one of two conclusions. The first is that education directly causes good health. The second is that longer education produces some effect in people that helps them take better care of their health. Given the earlier conclusion that the cause of health inequality is unhealthy behaviour, this seems to fit. People with more education learn better how to adopt healthy lifestyles and make better use of health services.

A more sophisticated version of this argument would be that education equips people better to make the trade-offs between having more fun now (sex and drugs and rock 'n roll) and investing in their future. Or that education helps people get a grip on their own lives and environment – and end up healthier as a result.

One UK study found that each Civil Service grade had worse health in terms of heart and circulation than the one above it.[24] This led the researchers to suggest people with little control over their lives at work were less likely to adopt healthy practices and might be under extra pressure at work that could bring on heart attacks. A more convincing explanation would be that people who ended up in such jobs did so because they lacked the educational qualifications that would also have helped them get better control of their health.

The role of government

To sum up, there appears to be growing health inequality in Britain where those in the lowest classes suffer worse health than those at the top of the ladder. Partly this can be explained by the great improvement in the condition of the healthiest sections of society. But it can also be explained by the persistence in less healthy behaviour such as smoking and other forms of over-indulgence which carries people off prematurely.

People can change their behaviour quite quickly, which is why some groups have succeeded in making rapid improvements in their life-chances. But other groups find it harder to change their behaviour – and the reason appears to be poor education. Merely giving people more money would be unlikely to have much impact on their health.

None of these facts means that government can step back from the issue of health inequality. Indeed, it is only the government that can affect the primary cause of the differentials, through the education system. But given that it takes time to change the education system – and two-thirds of the population has passed beyond its reach – what then can government do to improve the health of the most disadvantaged groups?

The simple answer is to continue with what has been happening since 1992, when the last Conservative government launched *The Health of the Nation,* a white paper on reducing preventable illnesses and encouraging healthy behaviour.[25] This aimed to reduce illness in five 'key areas': coronary heart disease and stroke, cancers, mental illness, accidents and HIV/AIDS and sexual health. To achieve this, it set targets for reducing four risk factors: smoking, bad diet, high blood pressure and needle-sharing among drug misusers. Health authorities were encouraged to draw up strategies to achieve the targets, and progress was regularly reviewed by Whitehall.

At first, there was considerable scepticism over some of the targets. Many seemed to have been chosen by projecting forward well-established trends – allowing the government to claim success for doing nothing but waiting. In fact this turned out to be optimistic and within a few years, several of the targets began to look unattainable. Progress has been made in some areas, such as reducing accidents, heart disease and breast cancer. But on obesity, female drinking and teenage smoking, incidence is rising – all factors where personal behaviour needs to change.[26]

The Labour government has maintained the idea of targets in *Our Healthier Nation,* its green paper published in early 1998.[27] However, it reduced the key areas to four by removing HIV/AIDS and sexual diseases. It also set fewer targets overall, saying this would give greater flexibility for health authorities to address local problems and tackle inequality. No firm targets were set on reducing inequality, though local policymakers will be required to set them.

It is clear that achieving any of the targets on the four key areas will require a concerted – and focused – attack on forms of behaviour that threaten the health of particular groups. Ingenuity will be needed in finding ways to change consumption patterns. And one promising approach is to pay people to behave better – which a recent survey of eleven trials carried out with appropriate controls found had produced good results in ten.[28]

Some of the experiments involved paying small sums to low-income patients or the homeless to turn up for appointments with dentists, post-natal clinics or anti-tuberculosis drives. Others offered money to those who met weight-loss targets, reduced their blood pressure by taking the appropriate drugs or stayed off cocaine. Financial incentives generally worked better than alternatives such as sending reminders or asking friends to help which also cost more.

Having health services free at the point of use may make it easier for people at risk to see doctors. If they drop in to a surgery when they are worried about an aspect of their health or when they have a minor ailment, their GP has an opportunity to screen them and discuss health issues. But this is a haphazard way of targeting those who suffer from health inequality who – by definition – are already losing out from a free health service.

If the government is serious about reducing health inequality, it needs a pro-active approach that seeks out those most at risk and helps them change their unhealthy behaviour. Free health services help those who already know how to help themselves. Charging where it can be afforded allows the NHS to increase the size of its budget and provide more for its patients. But it would also provide resources for making the only form of attack on health inequality that is likely to work: targeted campaigns aimed at those who already slip through the net.

10: Prescription for Recovery

The National Health Service has reached its half-century in a world vastly different to that in which it was conceived and born. In many ways, it has survived better than might have been expected at various crisis points in its history. And it could well survive another 50 years – at least in name.

But if the NHS does carry on to its centenary, it will suffer all the difficulties faced by the elderly in a rapidly changing world. New and more nimble alternatives will spring up – such as the walk-in medical centres mentioned in Chapter 7. The rather lumbering private medical insurance sector which barely poses a threat today will develop new and more attractive products. The health service will find itself increasingly out of tune with the demands of a society in which people are less prepared to accept they cannot have something that is well within their financial reach.

Remember that the UK is already three times richer than when Bevan launched his free, state-financed health service. Then life was still a struggle for most working people, and universal benefits such as family allowances made the difference between poverty and a decent standard of living. Rationing to a degree that most young people today would find staggering was accepted – not least because it provided better nutrition for the majority of the population than at any time in history.

Home ownership was for a minority; 40 per cent of homes had no bathroom; cars were owned by a privileged few; foreign holidays unknown; most homes sparsely furnished and devoid of the appliances which are now enjoyed by more than 90 per cent of households. In such a society, providing health care free at the point of use was a good way to ensure it reached most people. And the vast majority of the population was happy to queue for a service that offered them far better treatment than before.

Today, it is only the health service that is rationed in Britain. Even those in the bottom 20 per cent of households enjoy standards of living that would seem quite luxurious to the average working class family of the late 1940s. Housing free of damp, central heating, proper bathrooms, cookers, washing machines, refrigerators, freezers, telephones, televisions and videos are all to be found in more than 75 per cent of the homes of those in the bottom fifth of the income distribution.[1]

The people in the bottom fifth spend almost £5 a week on tobacco; £3.60 on alcoholic drinks; £4.30 on leisure goods such as newspapers, electronic equipment and gardening supplies; and £10.35 on leisure services such as holidays, gambling and entertainment.[2] Nearly half own a car or van. Such figures are enough to suggest that modest charging for health care would be affordable, even in these lowest-income households. For the population as a whole, less modest charges can hardly be described as a threat to either health or general prosperity.

There is no reason to believe that the scale of change will be any less in the next 50 years. By the NHS's centenary, therefore, Britain will be three times wealthier than today – a society in which to ration health care by queuing will be even more irrational. Relatively expensive forms of treatment, by today's standards, would be within reach of most households.

That is not to say the NHS must inevitably pass on before

that point is reached. It is quite plausible it will continue in much of its present form – particularly if the Labour government succeeds in finding savings elsewhere in public spending to allow a boost in the share of GDP that goes into the health service. The Conservatives, after all, raised health spending as a proportion of GDP by one percentage point – 20 per cent – between 1985 and 1993.[3]

But it is equally plausible that by its centenary, the NHS will have become what its supporters have always opposed – a second-class service for those who cannot afford to pay for their own health care. Private health insurance now covers 13 per cent of the population, twice the proportion in 1980. At that rate of growth, it will be a long time before half the population is covered. Sooner than that, however, there will come a point when private insurance moves from being seen as a luxury to a necessity. The growth rate will then accelerate – as it did with goods such as cars, telephones, videos and personal computers.

If it is true that wealthier societies spend more on merit goods such as health care, increasing numbers will start to spend their own money on treatment. They are already doing so in all sorts of ways as we saw in Chapter 7, from alternative therapies to over-the-counter medicines. The Henley Centre found in 1997 that 37 per cent of people were prepared to pay for a guaranteed higher level of service from their GP. The 27 per cent willing to pay for regular visits were prepared to shell out an average of £9 a visit.[4]

None of this will eliminate the need for some sort of collective provision of health services to pay for the treatments which none but the wealthiest can afford. The risk of serious illness, catastrophic accidents and epidemics needs to be pooled in some way – through a National Health Service, social insurance funds such as are found in much of continental Europe or compulsory private insurance. Given that we have the NHS, it would be foolish to swap to an alternative such as private insurance with all its drawbacks. So long as the health service retains 'membership' of most of the population, it is an efficient and well-understood method of pooling risk.

But there lies the danger for the NHS: a loss of membership as people drift out of it and into private insurance. Those people will inevitably be the more affluent and healthiest in society, leaving the health service as a rump insurer for those who are too poor or unhealthy to take out private cover. If the NHS is to avoid this unappealing fate, it must adapt to provide the service that people want. Only by recognising the changing nature of British society can the health service keep the job it does best: pooling the health risks for the entire British population.

A future that works

If the National Health Service is to hold on to its franchise as health insurer to the British people, it must offer people a service they can be proud of. Whatever the warm feelings expressed about the NHS, it is far from achieving that goal. Britain deserves better – but it will need much more money to raise the standards, and a different relationship between the doctor and patient. While the NHS can never be entirely like Rudolf Klein's garage, it needs to be much more like one and a great deal less like a church.

There may be some scope over the next few years to raise public spending on the NHS. The government hopes to make savings from its social security reforms that can be ploughed into health and education. This dividend from the New Deal will be slow to come, however, and so far health spending has fallen behind the 3 per cent a year real increase averaged in previous decades.

A Whitehall review is looking at alternative ways of financing the health service, ground that has been well-trodden over the last 50 years. One path it will have to retread is the idea of a dedicated health tax – rather like national insurance contributions which are a form of dedicated pensions tax. There are many attractions to such an approach, since it might help overcome resistance to higher taxes. Taxpayers are legitimately worried that higher taxes destined for improvements in particular services disappear into a common pot and they rarely see the benefits. A dedicated health tax would mean that 'what you see is what you get'; it could be made subject to a ballot, allowing people to vote for higher spending on health care.

The disadvantages of such taxes are equally well-rehearsed. The amount collected will be linked to income or spending and thus will fluctuate with the economic cycle. If it is topped up by the Treasury – as the National Insurance Fund is – transparency is lost and the exercise begins to look like creative accountancy to raise taxes. The history of 'hypothecated taxes' is not encouraging either – the road fund tax is not used to build roads any more and simply boosts Treasury receipts.

In any case, the argument in favour of asking people to

pay is not simply one of bringing in more money – necessary though that is. It is about giving patients more choice, diversity and control over their health care spending, something the 1991 reforms failed to do. One of the Conservative government's favourite slogans in introducing the reforms was that the money would follow the patients. In fact, it is the patients who must follow the money, when they go for treatment with hospitals under the contracts drawn up by their health authority or fundholding GP.

The question of where treatment is given is, of course, only one small aspect of patient choice. Others include timing – when it is convenient to be seen by a GP or a good time to have a non-urgent operation. Then there is the range of treatments on offer, or the place where they are delivered, or the environment within which they are delivered.

All patients have similar needs at the onset of emergency and life-threatening conditions, but much health care – including recovery after treatment – falls in neither category. Some patients will rate factors such as convenience, speed, pleasant surroundings and so on as more important than others. As in so many other parts of everyday life, we all have different priorities – and some people are happy to pay for a higher level of luxury or convenience.

There are quite large parts of the health care sector where patients already exercise considerable choice. These include dentistry, now largely private for adults, and over-the-counter medicines. In both cases, people pay close to a market rate for treatment and decide for themselves whether the result is worth their marginal pound.

The same is true in the fast-growing sphere of alternative

medicine — osteopathy, homeopathy, acupuncture and the like. While some of this is becoming available on the NHS, these disciplines have mushroomed independently of it. Patients make their own decisions about paying the fees, and while critics may see them as foolish on the grounds that the therapies are ineffective, no one has yet suggested they should be stopped on the grounds of equity.

In fact, we already expect patients to make choices on non-cost issues in most aspects of medicine. The most important of these is giving consent for treatment, often involving complex issues where the risks are finely balanced. Parents, spouses and children can all find themselves weighing fundamental questions about the continuation of treatment against whether to let nature take its course.

It is not that people like to be consulted on such questions: they are *required* to express an opinion as part of ethical medical procedure. Why, then, should not the thinking patient who can be trusted to make these life-and-death decisions also be given a role when it comes to other aspects of health care — such as the where, when, what and who of treatment?

At the moment, the patient is a passive recipient of the treatment allocated by the doctor, health authority or trust. It might suit the patient to pay a little extra to adjust the one-size-fits-all product given away in the NHS — to have an appointment at a convenient time, for example, or fit in a non-urgent operation during a lull at work. But there is no such provision, and nor can there be in the present system because the patient's preferences are deemed worthless or damaging to the interests of others who may have different preferences.

That is why sooner or later, more people will decide to pay for more of their health care. Not just because it will get them better treatment faster, but because it will give them more of a say in what they get. Whether or not this is a good thing is, in one sense, irrelevant (though I happen to think it is good – a symptom of the progress made in raising the standards and expectations of British people). It is already happening and it will happen more in the future.

And because of the benefits that can be engineered from allowing people to pay something towards their health care, it should be welcomed. More money and positive choices means less waste and diminished rationing. And the additional funds can be used to tackle the inequalities which the free NHS fails to address.

A charging package

Paying to visit an osteopath or for a packet of painkillers may be on the increase, but most people will find it a big jump to start paying to see a doctor or for hospital treatment. That is one reason why charging should involve modest amounts, initially at least. If the charges look comparable to the amounts people pay for a meal in a fast-food restaurant or a round in a pub, they are likely to prove more acceptable than a large lump sum or insurance premium.

At the same time, the charges should not be too low, or they will be swallowed up by the cost of collection. Putting in payment systems will be an expensive one-off expense in introducing charging, and the investment must be seen to be worthwhile straightaway.

PRESCRIPTION FOR RECOVERY

That suggests a charging package along the lines set out in Chapter 7:

- a fee for seeing a doctor, whether GP or hospital physician, of £10 a time – this would raise £3.3 billion before exemptions
- increasing the number of people who pay prescription charges by restricting exemptions to those on means-tested benefits – bringing in more than £800 million a year
- a charge for using hospitals of £25 for day surgery and £50 for a longer stay, with only one charge in any twelve-month period to avoid overtaxing the sick or disabled – raising £300 million a year
- additional charges for special hospital services such as single rooms, guaranteed treatment dates and choice over time and date
- published tariffs for the more common elective operations such as hip replacements and cataract surgery, making it easier for people to go privately rather than wait – and releasing resources for those unable to pay.

Overall, the guesstimate is that this package could add up to £5 billion to the NHS budget, an increase of 10 per cent. Later, charges could be introduced for non-emergency surgery, as happens already with dentistry. Patients would pay a per-centage of the cost up to a certain limit such as £250 or £500 (and then not pay the hospital charge mentioned above).

The total raised would be reduced if there was an exten-sive system of exemptions. But as with prescription charges, the intention would be to minimise the numbers of people not paying. Restricting exemptions to those on means-tested benefits would have the advantage of simplicity, especially if the government goes ahead with the introduction of an identity card system for those entitled to free benefits.

Households on means-tested benefits will include many pensioners and people with children. But there is no rationale for extending exemption to all pensioners or all children – or for continuing those exemptions which currently exist for these two groups. Many pensioners are well over the income limits for means-tested benefits, and 20 per cent have incomes above the average for society as a whole. And children are more or less equally distributed through the income distribution – they are as likely to be in households above average income as below.

To help those who are not exempt, however, the amount paid in charges could be capped by extending the current season ticket system for prescriptions. This gives a year of free prescriptions in return for a single payment – £80.50 in 1997-98. Similar schemes could be introduced for doctors' and dentists' charges, with the option of a single payment to cover all three sets of charges. This would stop people staying away from the doctor because they feared a continuing drain on their resources. It would be particularly useful for people with chronic illnesses – only some of whom currently get free prescriptions under the rather haphazard set of exemptions.

So, for example, an individual might be able to cover all routine NHS charges including prescriptions for, say, £150 a year – £3 a week. A family rate might be set at £400 a year where there were two parents, rather less for one. The scheme would not cover treatment that followed over a certain cost, but would ensure that patients could make their initial consultations for a predictable charge.

And if an identity card scheme was not in place for people on means-tested benefits, the season ticket could be given to them free. Better still, it could be sold to them at a discount to emphasise that everyone pays and is entitled to be treated equally. Benefits could be boosted to compensate, and the fact that the season ticket lasted for a year would mean no sudden increase in costs on coming off benefits.

Tackling the inequalities

Ensuring that no one loses out from the introduction of charging is an impossible task – someone is bound to slip through the net. It will therefore be important to remember that one aim of asking patients to pay is to produce resources for a determined attack on health inequalities. It is the middle classes who get the most benefit from the free NHS which fails to reach those further down the ladder. The way to tackle those inequalities is through positive action aimed at those most at risk.

For example, screening programmes for high blood pressure appear to be effective in catching people who would otherwise avoid seeing a doctor. Similarly, free eye tests and dental check-ups can be targeted towards those who might be reluctant to pay. Campaigns could be aimed at particular communities such as inner-city housing estates, or groups of people at risk – such as those working in low-income workplaces, retired people and single parents. The Afro-Caribbean community is particularly at risk from glaucoma and thus a targeted screening programme for that condition would be useful.

The success of such targeted initiatives will depend on the use of innovative marketing skills. Mobile clinics should be made to look as inviting as the stands that promote consumer products in shopping centres. They should be sent out to places where the target audience can be found – drop-in centres for the elderly, refuges for the homeless, outside schools and so on.

All the techniques used in new product launches should be considered. One of these is offering vouchers – an approach already used in Sweden to reach groups who might be deterred by charges. Elderly and disabled patients were given vouchers to pay for taxis to get to and from hospitals, with a similar scheme introduced for dental services.[5]

Considerable care is needed to monitor such schemes: in Sweden taxi drivers began to ask for two vouchers per trip, for example, and there were allegations of vouchers being sold at a discount on a newly created black market – something that has afflicted the US food stamp programmes. There were also stories that some dentists were offering bottles of whisky in return for the vouchers of people needing no treatment. But such practices are inevitable if patients are given the resources to buy their own health care – and can be kept under control by effective monitoring.

Another way to reach those who fail to use the health service is direct contact by mail, telephone or in person. One study in the London Borough of Newham managed to double the number of women from ethnic minorities attending breast cancer screening by telephoning them or sending personalised letters. All it took was two hours' training in how to approach the target patients, a determined campaign and appropriate follow-up after the initial contact.[6]

At the same time, a taskforce should be created to target those patients who might suffer from the introduction of charges. The RAND study described in Chapter 8 suggests that this is a small minority, and many of those are currently losing out even in a free health service. The taskforce would be required to monitor health inequalities, explore the causes and devise programmes to deal with them.

A responsive health service

So far, little has been said about the structure of the NHS. The constant revolution of the past two decades suggests further reorganisations are unlikely to produce great improvements under the present system of funding health care. But an infusion of more money from charges is also likely to change relationships in the NHS, putting pressure on doctors and hospitals to respond more to patient needs – to become more like a garage, in other words. Structural changes could then help health care professionals and organisations become more responsive to patients.

Creating that responsiveness means encouraging diversity to meet patients' differing needs. The best way to promote such diversity is by fostering benign competition, so health care organisations can experiment to see what it is that patients really want. Sadly, the idea of competition in the NHS is not popular with the Labour government, which sees it as a source of variation in the way patients are treated as well as a waste of resources that creates needless duplication.[7]

The irony about worries over variation in treatment caused by competition is that there is already considerable variation across the NHS. As we saw in Chapter 1, the differences in the treatment levels offered by health authorities are greater than can be explained by need. The variations between different parts of the country, however, are much less visible than those created by competition locally – as can be seen from the criticism of fundholding that it creates a two-tier NHS. As one observer puts it: 'Instead of the unknown wait in bus queues in another area, a taxi now stops and picks up selected people from the same queue in full view of those remaining.'[8]

So long as the differences introduced by competition represent improvements on what was previously available, this is defensible. The answer to a patient who says his or her doctor is offering a lower standard of service than another is not to force everyone to have the same poor service: it is to extend the improvements to everyone. Patients can help in the process by asking their own doctors why they are not offering as good a service as another.

Clearly there are limits to this argument: variation could leave some people worse off if their doctors prove incompetent in adapting to change and there are no alternative doctors in the area. This is often the case in inner-city areas where the family doctor service is provided by single GPs practising from lock-up shops with little threat of competition from better-run practices. But while there is a real problem here, it is not insuperable if properly addressed and carefully monitored. Failing doctors should be replaced or bolstered with additional resources as has already happened with schools – not left offering a poor service to those who most need the NHS.

As for the waste involved in competition, there have certainly been some egregious examples in the NHS – usually because managers unused to the private sector have been encouraged to behave like captains of industry. The result has been the sort of expensive rebranding and proliferation of logos which gave the 1991 reforms a bad name.

But the experience in most other walks of life is that any extra costs of competition are usually outweighed by the savings from the greater efficiency of meeting the needs of consumers effectively. In the NHS, for example, the cost of not meeting patients' needs can be seen in the £500 million a year it costs the NHS when patients fail to turn up for appointments and operations.[9] Good customer-responsive industries have learnt that it is not fearsome price-cutting which delivers commercial success: it is meeting the needs of their customers at prices they can afford.

Alain Enthoven, the US academic who drew up the original blueprint for the internal market, identified the lack of incentives to meet the patient's needs as a key weakness of the health service. There were, he wrote in 1985, 'no serious incentives to guide the NHS in the direction of better quality care and service at reduced cost'.[10] That remains substantially the position, as we saw in Chapter 4.

Creating those 'serious incentives' can be done in only one way: opening up competition, rather than reducing it. No one believes that less competition in any other sector of life would improve services – and the same is true in health care. Competition could be increased in all three parts of the NHS as currently constituted without leading to disastrous consequences.

First, the health authorities which buy health care on behalf of the people who live in their areas. Although their creation marked the break-up of the monolithic health service run directly from Whitehall, they are still local monopolies – like the old electricity boards. There is no reason why they should not be allowed to compete in each others areas, signing up patients and organising their health services in return for a bigger share of the NHS budget. Most people would stick with their local health authority, but some would begin to swap and that would put pressure on the authorities to be more responsive to patients. A health authority that proved successful in organising shorter waiting lists, for example, would pick up patients from others, which would then be forced to follow suit.

There is already nominally competition between hospitals and trusts – but this is far from the reality in practice, as we saw in Chapter 4. In many parts of the country, there is only one large district general hospital which can provide the full range of services within easy reach. Some way needs to be found to introduce competition into these large institutions.

One example of how local monopolies can be opened to competition is airports and shopping malls. Inside these buildings, many businesses compete – whether it be shops, restaurants, baggage handlers, car-hire firms or whatever. It would be quite possible for a large hospital to function in a similar way – providing a building and facilities for different 'firms' of medical professionals to offer their services.

Thus various surgical teams would use the same hospital, working with other 'firms' which would provide anaesthetics, diagnostic services, aftercare and so on. In practice large hospitals tend to work in this way anyway, coordinating these various functions. The difference would be to encourage more than one team in some areas, so doctors and surgeons could compete for patients by offering better services.

This might seem impossibly complex to administer, except that it is often what happens in the private sector of medicine. And large professional service firms such as lawyers, accountants and consultants effectively operate in such a way, assembling appropriate teams for particular assignments. In industries such as information technology and software, 'virtual firms' are emerging which bring together independent workers for individual projects. Health services will do the same sooner or later, to the benefit of patients.

The third element of the NHS is the GP fundholders, about to be abolished by the new government. While fundholding has produced fewer benefits for patients than might have been expected, it has been a source of innovation. And Frank Dobson, Labour's Health Secretary, has recognised the benefits of giving GPs a bigger role with his move to introduce locality commissioning for family doctors. This will group GPs in each area and give them the budget to buy services within guidelines set by the district health authority.

Locality commissioning has already been piloted by district health authorities concerned at the reduction in their budgets caused by the growth of fundholding. Its benefits have yet to be proved, however. A study of locality commissioning in Avon found improvements in patients' access to services and better cooperation between practices. But the impact was largely felt in primary care and community services rather than in the hospital services where the bulk of NHS costs fall.

Most of the doctors involved felt they had had little influence on the health authority. And there were signs that the enthusiasm of participants – key to its success – could wane without more resources to manage the scheme. Overall, there was frustration that the scheme relied on the efforts of the most motivated, leaving others doing comparatively little.

Locality commissioning is a good way to involve smaller practices which are not large enough to act as fundholders in buying services for their patients. From the point of view of the patient, however, it might be better to see the gradual disappearance of the smaller practices. Their replacement by larger health centres controlling their own budgets could mean a much greater range of health services closer to the patient that would also be cheaper than hospital treatment.

Selling the unthinkable

Charges for treatment, fewer exemptions, more competition to stimulate innovation – none of this would be easy to sell to the public, whatever the dissatisfaction with the status quo. Voters distrust politicians interfering in the NHS, are loyal to their local hospitals and doctors, and fear change will lead to American-style insecurity.

The experience of the Conservatives in the 1991 reforms is not encouraging. Their white paper *Working For Patients* took a bullish approach to selling the changes, no doubt be-

cause its authors knew they were doing nothing to undermine the basic principles of the National Health Service.
They restated those principles and set out an agenda which
committed the government to improving the health service:

- The NHS is, and will continue to be, open to all,
  regardless of income, and financed mainly out of general
  taxation.
- The Government wants to raise the performance of all
  hospitals and GP practices to that of the best.[11]

The twin aims of the proposals were to give patients 'greater
choice of the services available' and to secure 'greater satisfaction and rewards for those working in the NHS who successfully respond to local needs and preferences'. Who could
possibly disagree with such aims? It quickly turned out that
almost everyone did. *Working for Patients* sparked the most fe-
rocious debate in the NHS since its foundation.[12]

The opposition was intensified by several specific factors:
generalised hostility to Mrs Thatcher (this was the era of the
poll tax, and came just before her downfall); the peremptory
nature of the review; the stance of Kenneth Clarke, the rum-
bustious Health Secretary who had already forced through
education reforms in the teeth of opposition from teachers;
the government's determination to force through the reforms against opposition without conceding, for example, a
pilot study; a degree of political opportunism by the opposition.

But in case anyone should think there is any greater public realism about the need for change in the health service,

the MORI poll carried out for the Social Market Foundation in summer 1997 makes clear the opposition to charging. Two-thirds of those questioned believed the NHS should be free for everyone at the point of use.[13]

That finding was perhaps predictable: a free service always seems attractive. Other parts of the survey suggest the line of argument that would be most persuasive in changing public opinion. Two-thirds thought the NHS would have to cut back its services over the next ten years, and four out of five were opposed to any such reduction.[14] Stressing that charges would generate the income to avoid cuts might make them more palatable to the public.

Roger Douglas, the finance minister in New Zealand's re-forming Labour government of the 1980s, emphasises that change can be made politically popular if the benefits to voters are clearly set out: 'Winning public acceptance depends on demonstrating that you are improving opportunities for the nation as a whole while protecting the most vulnerable groups in the community.'[15]

A programme to reform the National Health Service must start from the conviction that the present arrangements are not the best in the world, and that they fall far short of what Britain deserves. It must demonstrate to voters that the proposed charges will improve health services for everyone. It should emphasise that charging is used in almost every other advanced country – many of which have better health services. And the risks of change must be contrasted with the shortfalls in the present NHS which deny treatment to those who need it.

If the health service can be renewed to reflect the fast-changing world in which it now finds itself, it can enjoy a second half-century as exciting as its first 50 years. The hardest part of that renewal will be to realise that preserving one of the NHS's fundamental values – a universal service – can be achieved only by sacrificing another – free at the point of use.

A free service was an essential feature at the birth of the National Health Service in the peculiar circumstances of post-war reconstruction. Today it looks anachronistic and is debilitating in its consequences. But a universal health service which retains the membership of the vast majority of people in Britain remains as valuable for social cohesion and improving the nation's health as it was 50 years ago. It is certainly worth struggling for.

Notes

Introduction

1 Rudolf Klein, *The New Politics of the NHS*, 1995, p. 229.

Chapter 1: A Health Service to be Proud of?

1 Henley Centre, *Planning for Social Change 1998*, 1997.
2 Geoffrey Rivett, *From Cradle to Grave: Fifty Years of the NHS*, 1998.
3 Lindsay Brook, John Hall and Ian Preston, 'Public Spending and Taxation' in Roger Jowell et al (eds.), *British Social Attitudes – The 13th Report*, 1996, p. 186.
4 Elias Mossialos, 'Citizens' Views on Healthcare Systems in the 15 Member States of the European Union', *Health Economics*, vol. 6, 1997, pp. 109-116.
5 Martin Powell, *Evaluating the National Health Service*, 1997, pp. 160, 179.
6 Sean Boyle and Anthony Harrison, 'The Management of Emergency Care: Who Is Responsible?', in Anthony Harrison (ed.), *Healthcare UK 1995/96*, 1996, p. 165.
7 Henry Aaron and W. B. Schwartz, *The Painful Prescription: Rationing Hospital Care*, 1984, p. 101.
8 Bill New and Nicholas Mays, 'Age, renal replacement therapy and rationing', in Anthony Harrison and Bill New (eds.), *Healthcare UK 1996/97*, 1997, p. 206.
9 Sharon Kingman, 'Renal Services in UK are Underfunded, says Report', *BMJ*, vol. 312, 3 February 1996, p. 267.
10 Nick Bosanquet and Stephen Pollard, *Ready for Treatment*, 1997, p. 32.
11 R.M. Plowman, N. Graves & J.A. Roberts, *Hospital-Acquired Infection*, Office of Health Economics, 1997.
12 Naaz Coker, 'Smoke and Dust', *Health Service Journal*, 17 July 1997, p. 29.

13 John Edwards, 'Measuring the wasteline', *Health Service Journal,* 13 November 1997, pp. 26–27.

14 Consumers' Association, 'Hospital Care', *Which?,* August 1997, pp. 21–23.

15 Audit Commission, *Improving Your Image: How to Manage Radiology Services More Effectively,* 1995, p. 42.

16 Ibid. p. 15.

17 Audit Commission, *Goods for Your Health: Improving Supplies Management in NHS Trusts,* 1996, p. 8.

18 Ibid. p. 33.

19 Ibid. p. 12.

20 Ibid. p. 22.

21 Ibid. p. 28.

22 Ibid. p. 41.

23 Ibid. p. 55.

24 Audit Commission, *By Accident or Design: Improving A&E Services in England and Wales,* 1996, p. 11.

25 Anthony Harrison and Bill New, *Healthcare UK 1995/96,* 1997, p. 49.

26 The hospital league tables were published on the internet in July 1997 at www.open.gov.uk/doh/tables97/index.htm.

27 Audit Commission, *By Accident or Design,* 1996, p. 12.

28 Speech to the Association of Community Health Councils, Department of Health press notice 97/162, 9 July 1997.

29 Audit Commission, *By Accident or Design,* 1996, p. 14.

30 Ibid. p. 18.

31 Ibid. p. 51.

32 Secretary of State for Health, *The New NHS,* 1997, p. 42.

33 Harrison and New, *Healthcare UK 1996/97,* 1997, p. 8.

34 Efficiency Scrutiny Team, *Prescription Fraud: An Efficiency Scrutiny,* 1997, p. 34.

35 Jenny Griffiths, 'The Battle for the Future of Healthcare', in Sholom Glouberman (ed.), *Beyond Restructuring,* 1996, p. 98.

36 Sean Boyle and Richard Hamblin, *The Health Economy of London,* 1997, pp. 201ff.

37 Efficiency Scrutiny Team, 1997, p. 41.

38 Ibid. p. 55.

39 National Association of Health Authorities and Trusts, *Health and the Economy,* 1994.

40 NHS *Provides Good Value For Money Compared With Other Healthcare Systems,* Department of Health press notice 94/360, 28 July 1994.
41 *Daily Telegraph,* 21 January 1998.
42 Rudolf Klein, *The New Politics of the NHS,* 1995, p. 248.

Chapter 2: A Child of Scarcity

1 Rudolf Klein, Patricia Day and Sharon Redmayne, *Managing Scarcity: Priority Setting and Rationing in the National Health Service,* 1996, p. 37.
2 Rudolf Klein, *The New Politics of the NHS,* 1995, p. 248.
3 Nicholas Timmins, *The Five Giants: A Biography of the Welfare State,* 1995, p. 103.
4 Klein, *New Politics,* 1995, p. 4.
5 Timmins, *Five Giants,* 1995, p. 109.
6 Quoted in Klein, *New Politics,* 1995, p. 9.
7 Peter Hennessy, *Never Again: Britain 1945–1951,* 1992, p. 143.
8 Timmins, *Five Giants,* 1995, p. 128.
9 Ibid. p. 131.
10 Ibid. p. 18.
11 Hennessy, 1992, p. 73.
12 Correlli Barnett, *The Lost Victory: British Dreams, British Realities 1945–1950,* 1995, p. 129.
13 Timmins, *Five Giants,* 1995, p. 21.
14 Quoted in Hennessy, 1992, p. 38.
15 Barnett, 1995, p. 31.
16 Hennessy, 1992, p. 76ff.
17 Charles Webster, *The Health Services Since the War,* 1988, p. 133.
18 Quoted in Barnett, 1995, p. 143.
19 Webster, 1988, Table 1.
20 Timmins, *Five Giants,* 1995, p. 158.
21 Ibid. p. 130.
22 Quoted in Hennessy, 1992, p. 50.
23 Ibid. p. 51.
24 Ibid. p. 89.
25 Ibid. p. 315–16.
26 Ibid. p. 128.
27 Sholom Glouberman (ed.), *Beyond Restructuring: A Collection of Papers from a King's Fund International Seminar,* 1996, p. 11.

28 Klein, *New Politics*, 1995, pp. 28ff.

29 Ibid. p. 61.

30 Ibid. p. 36.

31 John Yates, *Why Are We Waiting? An Analysis of Hospital Waiting Lists*, 1987, p. 2.

32 Martin Powell, *Evaluating the National Health Service*, 1997, p. 113.

33 Klein, *New Politics*, 1995, pp. 47ff.

34 Ibid. p. 33.

35 Nicholas Timmins, *Financial Times,* 5 July 1997.

36 Jon Hibbs, *Daily Telegraph,* 7 August 1997.

37 Klein, *New Politics*, 1995, p. 142.

38 Glouberman (ed.), 1996, p. 13.

39 Klein, *New Politics*, 1995, p. 50.

40 Ibid. p. 101.

41 Office of Health Economics, *Compendium of Health Statistics*, 1997, Table 2.7.

42 Klein, *New Politics*, 1995, p. 69.

43 Robert Maxwell, 'The Limits of Simple Fixes', in Glouberman (ed.), 1996, p. 139.

44 Roy Griffiths, NHS *Management Inquiry*, 1983.

45 Klein, *New Politics*, 1995, p. 150.

46 Nigel Lawson, *The View From No. 11,* 1992, p. 303.

47 House of Commons Social Services Committee, *Fourth Report, Session 1985–86, Public Expenditure on the Social Services*, HMSO, London, 1986, HC 387.

48 Reply to Social Services Committee First Report, Session 1987–88, vol. 11, pp. 96–108.

49 Nicholas Timmins, *Cash, Crisis and Cure,* 1988, pp. 31ff.

50 Nicholas Timmins, *Independent,* 9 December 1987.

51 Lawson, 1992, p. 612.

52 Timmins, *Cash, Crisis and Cure*, 1988, p. 44.

53 Ibid. p. 45.

Chapter 3: When Scarcity Ran Out

1 Rudolf Klein, *The New Politics of the NHS,* 1995, p. 133.

2 William Laing, *Laing's Review of Private Healthcare 1997,* 1997, Table 3.1.

3 Michael Calnan, Sarah Cant and Jonathan Gabe, *Going Private: Why People Pay For Their Healthcare,* 1993, p. 80.

4 Martin Powell, *Evaluating the National Health Service,* 1997, p. 84.

5 Replaced by Kenneth Clarke and David Mellor who became Health Secretary and Health Minister when the Department of Health and Social Security was split in July 1988.

6 Nigel Lawson, *The View From No. 11,* 1992, p. 614.

7 Nicholas Timmins, *The Five Giants: A Biography of the Welfare State,* 1995, p. 460. David Willetts subsequently became a Conservative MP.

8 Lawson, 1992, p. 616.

9 Quoted in Chris Ham, 'The United Kingdom', in Chris Ham (ed.), *Healthcare Reform – Learning from International Experience,* 1997, p. 47.

10 Alain Enthoven, *Reflections on the Management of the National Health Service,* 1985.

11 Timmins, *Five Giants,* 1995, p. 462.

12 Private information.

13 Secretaries of State for Health, Wales, Northern Ireland and Scotland, *Working For Patients,* 1989.

14 Klein, *New Politics,* 1995, p. 202.

15 Ibid. p. 195.

16 Enthoven, 1985, p. 29.

17 Ham, 1997, p. 52.

18 *NHS Chief Executive Welcomes 'Successful First Six Months For NHS Reforms',* Department of Health press notice 98/17, 14 January 1992.

19 *Largest Ever Drop In Long Waiting Times,* Department of Health press notice 92/69, 10 February 1992.

20 *New Survey Shows NHS Trusts Are More Popular with Patients,* Department of Health press notice 92/16, 14 January 1992.

21 Radical Statistics Health Group, 'NHS Indicators of "Success": What do they Tell Us?', *BMJ,* vol. 310, 1995, pp. 1045–50.

22 Julian Le Grand, 'Evaluating the NHS Reforms', in Ray Robinson and Julian Le Grand (eds.), *Evaluating the NHS Reforms,* 1993, p. 259.

23 Margaret Whitehead, Maria Evandrou, Bengt Haglund and Finn Diderichsen, 'As the Health Divide Widens in Sweden and Britain, What's Happening to Access to Care?', *BMJ,* vol. 315, 1997, pp. 1007–08.

24 Neil Söderlund, Ivan Csaba, Alastair Gray, Ruairidh Milne and James Rafferty, 'Impact of the NHS Reforms on English Hospital Productivity: An Analysis of the First Three Years', *BMJ,* vol. 315, 1997,

pp. 1126–29.

25 Clas Rehnberg, 'Sweden', in Chris Ham (ed.), *Healthcare Reform,* 1997, p. 82.

26 Anders Anell, 'Implementing Planned Markets in Health Services: The Swedish Case', in Richard Saltman & Casten von Otter (eds.), *Implementing Planned Markets in Healthcare*, 1995, p. 213.

27 Wynand van de Ven, 'The Netherlands', in Ham (ed.), *Healthcare Reform – Learning from International Experience,* 1997, p. 93.

28 Organisation for Economic Co-operation and Development, *The Reform of Healthcare: A Comparative Analysis of Seven OECD Countries,* 1992.

29 Julian Le Grand and Will Bartlett, *Quasi-Markets and Social Policy*, 1995.

30 Enthoven, 1985, p. 17.

31 Quoted in Peter Hennessy, *Never Again: Britain 1945–1951,* 1992, p. 132.

32 Nick Bosanquet and Stephen Pollard, *Ready for Treatment,* 1997, p. 60.

33 Calnan, Cant and Gabe, 1993, p. 80.

34 Nick Bosanquet, 'Improving Health', in Roger Jowell et al (eds.), *British Social Attitudes: The 11th Report,* 1994, p. 57.

35 *The Citizen's Charter – Raising the Standard,* Cm 1599, London, HMSO, July 1991.

36 Secretary of State for Health, *The Patient's Charter,* 1991.

37 Anthony Harrison and Bill New, 'Health Policy Review', in Anthony Harrison & Bill New (eds.), *Healthcare UK 1996/97,* 1997, p. 49. The 1997 figure was published with the hospital league tables on the internet at www.open.gov.uk/doh/tables97/index.htm.

38 NHS *On Course To Deliver New Patient's Charter Guarantee On Waiting Times,* Department of Health press notice 95/68, 14 February 1995.

39 Bosanquet, 'Improving Health', in Jowell et al (eds.), *British Social Attitudes: The 11th Report,* 1994.

40 Ken Judge and Michael Solomon, 'Public Opinion and the National Health Service: Patterns and Perspectives in Consumer Satisfaction', *Journal of Social Policy,* vol. 22(3), July 1993, pp. 302–04.

Chapter 4: Unfinished Business

1 Sharon Redmayne, Rudolf Klein and Patricia Day, *Sharing Out Resources: Purchasing and Priority Setting in the NHS,* 1993, p. 29.
2 Sharon Redmayne, *Small Steps, Big Goals: Purchasing Policies in the NHS,* 1996.
3 Cited in Anthony Harrison and Bill New, 'Health Policy Review', in Anthony Harrison and Bill New (eds.), *Healthcare UK 1996/97: An Annual review of Healthcare Policy,* 1997, p. 5.
4 Philip Milner – cited in Harrison and New, *Healthcare UK 1996/97,* 1997, p. 6.
5 Redmayne, *Small Steps,* 1996, p. 4.
6 Harrison and New (eds.), *Healthcare UK 1996/97,* 1997, p. 6.
7 Will Bartlett, 'Quasi-markets and contracts: a markets and hierarchies perspective on NHS Reform', *Public Money,* vol. 11(3), 1991, pp. 53–61.
8 Rudolf Klein, Patricia Day and Sharon Redmayne, *Managing Scarcity: Priority Setting and Rationing in the National Health Service,* 1996, p. 51.
9 *Guardian,* 10 July 1997.
10 Alan Maynard, 'Can Competition Enhance Efficiency in Health Care? Lessons from the Reform of the UK National Health Service', *Social Science and Medicine,* vol. 39(10), 1994, p. 1439.
11 William Fitzhugh, *The Fitzhugh Directory of NHS Trusts 1997,* London, Healthcare Information Services, 1997, p. 18.
12 Alain Enthoven, *Reflections on the Management of the National Health Service,* 1985, p. 9.
13 Anthony Harrison, *Healthcare UK 1994/95: An Annual Review of Healthcare Policy,* 1995, p. 156.
14 Audit Commission, *Goods For Your Health: Improving Supplies Management in NHS Trusts,* 1996, p. 48.
15 Enthoven, 1985, p. 13.
16 Quoted in Klein, Day and Redmayne, *Managing Scarcity,* 1996, p. 64.
17 Jenny Griffiths, 'The Battle for the Future of Healthcare', in Sholom Glouberman (ed.), *Beyond Restructuring,* 1996, p. 101.
18 Office of Health Economics, *Compendium of Health Statistics,* 1997, Table 3.26.
19 Anthony Harrison and Sally Prentice, *Acute Futures,* 1996, p. 131.
20 C. Chantler and A. Maynard, 'Should Trusts be Allowed to Fail?', *BMJ,* vol. 314, 1997, p. 1566.

21 Clive Smee, 'Self-governing Trusts and GP Fundholders: The British Experience', in Richard Saltman and Casten von Otter (eds.), *Implementing Planned Markets in Healthcare*, 1995, p. 205.

22 Rebecca Surender, Jean Bradlow, Angela Coulter, Helen Doll, Sarah Stewart Brown, 'Prospective Study of Trends in Referral Patterns in Fundholding and Non-Fundholding Practices in the Oxford Region, 1990–94', *BMJ*, vol. 311, 1995, pp. 1205-08.

23 Therese Rafferty, Keith Wilson-Davis and Hugh McGavock, 'How Has Fundholding in Northern Ireland Affected Prescribing Patterns? A Longitudinal Study', *BMJ*, vol. 315, 1997, p. 168.

24 Howard Glennerster, Manos Matsaganis, Pat Owens and Stephanie Hancock, 'GP Fundholding: Wild Card or Winning Hand?', in Robinson and Le Grand (eds.), *Evaluating the NHS Reforms*, 1993, p. 100.

25 David Colin-Thomé, *Why Fundholding Should Stay*, 1997, p. 11.

26 Secretary of State for Health, *The New NHS: Modern, Dependable*, 1997.

27 Nick Goodwin, 'GP Fundholding: a Review of the Evidence', in Anthony Harrison (ed.), *Healthcare UK 1995/96*, 1996, p. 122.

28 *Financial Times*, 19 July 1997.

29 Goodwin, 1996, p. 127.

30 Audit Commission, *What the Doctor Ordered: A Study of GP Fundholders in England and Wales*, 1996, p. 86.

31 Ibid. p. 7.

32 Maynard, 'Can Competition Enhance Efficiency in Healthcare?', 1994, p. 1437.

33 Robert Maxwell, 'The Limits of Simple Fixes', in Glouberman (ed.), 1996, p. 145.

Chapter 5: Paradise Postponed – The Coffers Empty

1 Nicholas Timmins, *Financial Times*, 18 October 1996.

2 *Provisional Waiting List Figures, 31 December 1997*, Department of Health press notice 98/065, 19 February 1998.

3 Nicholas Timmins, *Financial Times*, 3 July 1997.

4 Evidence to the Commons Social Services Select Committee, 1985–86, quoted in Rudolf Klein, *The New Politics of the NHS*, 1995, p. 179.

5 The following sections draw extensively on Sarah Wordsworth, Cam Donaldson and Anthony Scott, *Can We Afford the NHS?*, 1996.

6 Thomas Getzen, 'Population Ageing and the Growth of Health Expenditures', *Journal of Gerontology,* Social Sciences, vol. 47(3), 1992, p. S98.

7 Ibid. p. S102.

8 Mia Defever, 'Long-Term Care: The Case of the Elderly', *Health Policy,* vol. 19, 1991, p. 8.

9 Getzen, 1992, p. S98.

10 Defever, 1991, p. 12.

11 Gail Wilson, 'Models of Ageing and their Relation to Policy Formation and Service Provision', *Policy and Politics,* vol. 19(1), 1991, p. 44.

12 Anthony Harrison, Jennifer Dixon, Bill New and Ken Judge, 'Can the NHS Cope in Future?', *BMJ,* vol. 314, 1997, p. 139.

13 Office for National Statistics, *Living in Britain 1995,* London, The Stationery Office, 1997, Table 7.1.

14 Defever, 1991, p. 7.

15 Getzen, 1992, p. S103.

16 Office of Health Economics, *Compendium of Health Statistics,* 1997, Tables 3.25 and 3.26.

17 Ibid. Tables 3.21, 3.16.

18 Clive Cookson and Daniel Green, *Financial Times,* 30 October 1997.

19 Henry Aaron, 'Thinking about Healthcare Finance: Some Propositions', in Organisation for Economic Co-operation and Development, *Healthcare Reforms – The Will to Change,* 1996, p. 52.

20 Office for National Statistics, *Family Spending 1996–97,* London, The Stationery Office, 1997, Table 1.1.

21 Anna McCormick, John Charlton and Douglas Fleming, 'Who Sees Their General Practitioner and For What Reason?', *Health Trends,* vol. 27(2), pp. 34–35.

22 Secretary of State for Health, *The Patient's Charter,* 1991.

23 *Privacy And Dignity For Hospital Patients,* Department of Health press notice 97/19, 27 January 1997.

24 *Baroness Jay Announces New Drive To Rid The NHS of Mixed Sex Hospital Accommodation,* Department of Health press notice 97/190, 6 August 1997.

25 Quoted in Klein, *New Politics,* 1995, p. 151.

Chapter 6: Rationing is No Answer

1   Rudolf Klein, Patricia Day and Sharon Redmayne, *Managing Scarcity:
    Priority Setting and Rationing in the National Health Service,* 1996, p. 44.
2   Nicholas Timmins, *The Five Giants,* 1995, p. 259.
3   Klein, Day and Redmayne, *Managing Scarcity,* 1996, p. 41.
4   Martin Powell, *Evaluating the National Health Service,* 1997, p. 98.
5   Secretary of State for Health, *The Health of the Nation: A Strategy for
    Health in England,* 1992.
6   Stephen Harrison, 'Clinical Autonomy and Planned Markets: The
    British Case', in Richard Saltman and Casten von Otter (eds.),
    Implementing Planned Markets in Healthcare, 1995. p. 164.
7   Bill New and Julian Le Grand, *Rationing in the NHS: Principles and
    Pragmatism,* 1996, p. 16.
8   Klein, Day and Redmayne, *Managing Scarcity,* 1996, p. 69.
9   Karen Bloor, Alan Maynard and Nick Freemantle, 'Can expenditure
    on Drugs be Contained Efficiently?', in Anthony Harrison (ed.),
    Healthcare UK 1995/96, London, King's Fund, 1996, p. 175.
10 New and Le Grand, *Rationing in the NHS,* 1996, p. 12.
11 *Additions to the list of items which may not be supplied on NHS prescription,*
    Department of Health press notice 93/989, 11 October 1993.
12 Secretary of State for Health, *The New NHS: Modern, Dependable,* 1997,
    para. 1.18.
13 Klein, Day and Redmayne, *Managing Scarcity,* 1996, p. 72.
14 The following sections draw heavily on New and Le Grand, *Rationing
    in the NHS,* 1996.
15 Klein, Day and Redmayne, *Managing Scarcity,* 1996, p. 75.
16 Ibid. p. 39.
17 Ibid. p. 77. In the end, treatment was financed by a private benefactor.
    Despite initial success, Jaymee Bowen died in May 1996.
18 Nicholas Timmins, *Independent,* 2 January 1996.
19 Secretary of State for Health, *The New NHS,* 1997, para. 8.5(ii).
20 Ibid. para. 7.11.
21 Klein, Day and Redmayne, *Managing Scarcity,* 1996, p. 73.
22 New and Le Grand, *Rationing in the NHS,* 1996, p. 20.
23 Ibid. p. 1.
24 *Virginia Bottomley Spells Out Policy On NHS Treatment For Elderly People,*
    Department of Health press notice 94/182, 15 April 1994.

25 New and Le Grand, *Rationing in the NHS*, 1996, p. 20.

26 Klein, Day and Redmayne, *Managing Scarcity*, 1996, p. 76.

27 Judy Allsop, *Health Policy and the NHS*, 1995, p. 83.

28 New and Le Grand, *Rationing in the NHS*, 1996, p. 14.

29 Klein, Day and Redmayne, *Managing Scarcity*, 1996, p. 125.

30 Frank Honigsbaum, Stefan Holmström and Johan Calltorp, *Making Choices for Healthcare*, 1997, p. 107.

31 Nick Bosanquet and Stephen Pollard, *Ready for Treatment*, 1997, p. 62.

32 New and Le Grand, *Rationing in the NHS*, 1996, p. 59.

33 Klein, Day and Redmayne, *Managing Scarcity*, 1996, p. 33.

34 Ibid. p. 109.

35 Ibid. p. 111.

36 Honigsbaum, Holmström and Calltorp, 1997, p. 12.

37 Ibid. p. 36.

38 Klein, Day and Redmayne, *Managing Scarcity*, 1996, p. 117.

39 Honigsbaum, Holmström and Calltorp, 1997, p. 19.

40 Ibid. p. 50.

Chapter 7: The Real Crisis in the NHS

1   Nick Bosanquet and Stephen Pollard, *Ready for Treatment*, 1997, pp. 44, 48.

2   Big MacCurrencies, *The Economist*, vol. 343, 12 April 1997.

3   Martin Powell, *Evaluating the National Health Service*, 1997, p. 179.

4   Rudolf Klein, *The New Politics of the NHS*, 1995, p. 305.

5   Paul Belien, 'What Can Europe's Healthcare Systems Tell Us About the Market's Role?', in William McArthur, Celia Ramsay and Michael Walker (eds.), *Healthy Incentives: Canadian Health Reform in an International Context*, 1996, p. 46.

6   Göran Berleen, Clas Rehnberg and Gunnar Wennström, *The Reform of Healthcare in Sweden*, 1993.

7   Powell, 1997, p. 171.

8   Wynand van de Ven, 'The Netherlands', in Chris Ham (ed.), *Healthcare Reform – Learning from International Experience*, 1997, p. 91.

9   Powell, 1997, p. 164.

10 This section draws heavily on Howard Glennerster, *Paying for Welfare – Towards 2000*, 1997, Chapter 8; and Nicholas Barr, 'Economic Theory

and the Welfare State: A Survey and Interpretation', *Journal of Economic Literature,* vol. 30, June 1992, pp. 749ff.

11 Secretary of State for Health, *The New NHS: Modern, Dependable,* 1997, para. 1.18.

12 Glennerster, *Paying for Welfare*, 1997, p. 141.

13 William Hsiao, 'Marketisation – the Illusory Magic Pill', *Health Economics*, vol. 3, 1994, p. 355.

14 John Eversley and Charles Webster, 'Light on the Charge Brigade', *Health Service Journal,* 17 July 1997, p. 26.

15 Office of Health Economics, *Compendium of Health Statistics,* 1997, Tables 2.18, 2.19.

16 Eversley and Webster, 1997, p. 27.

17 Alan Earl-Slater, 'Privatising Medicines in the National Health Service', *Public Money and Management,* vol. 16, January–March 1996, p. 40.

18 Klein, *New Politics*, 1995, p. 35.

19 Eversley and Webster, 1997, p. 27.

20 NHS *To Reclaim Traffic Accident Missing Millions,* Department of Health press notice 97/378, 4 December 1997.

21 Stephen Bailey and Allan Bruce, 'Funding the National Health Service: The Continuing Search for Alternatives', *Journal of Social Policy,* vol. 23(4), October 1994, p. 503.

22 Proprietary Association of Great Britain, *Annual Report 1997,* London, PAGB, 1997, p. 20.

23 A. Blenkinsopp and C. Bradley, 'Over The Counter Drugs: Patients, Society and the Increase in Self-Medication', *BMJ*, vol. 312, 1996, p. 629.

24 Ibid. p. 630.

25 Ibid. p. 631.

26 Proprietary Association of Great Britain, 1997, p. 9.

27 Office for National Statistics, *Family Spending 1996–97,* London, The Stationery Office, 1997, Table 1.3.

28 Office of Health Economics, *Compendium of Health Statistics,* 1997, Tables 2.17, 2.23.

29 Bosanquet and Pollard, 1997, p. 64.

30 Ibid. p. 70.

31 Ibid. p. 64.

32 Ibid. p. 74.

33 Office for National Statistics, *Living in Britain 1995: General Household Survey,* London, The Stationery Office, 1997.

34 Department of Social Security, *Social Security Statistics 1997,* 1997, p. H303.

35 Office of Health Economics, 1997, Tables 3.20, 3.41.

36 Office for National Statistics, 1997. This figure is the aggregate of items 12.4 (TVs, videos, computers and audio equipment), 13.1 (Cinema and theatre), 13.2 (sports admissions and subscriptions), 13.3 (TV, video and satellite rental, television licences) and 13.4 (Miscellaneous entertainments).

37 Football Association Premier League, *National Fan Survey*, London, Football Association, 1998.

38 Bosanquet and Pollard, 1997, p. 72.

Chapter 8: Paying for Services

1 British Medical Association, *Options for Funding Healthcare,* London, BMA, October 1997, p. 17.

2 British Medical Association, *Financing the NHS: A Discussion Paper,* London, BMA, March 1996, p. 14.

3 Stephen Birch, 'Hypothesis: Charges to Patients Impair the Quality of Dental Care to Elderly People', *Age and Ageing,* vol. 18, 1989, p. 136.

4 Wynand van de Ven, 'Effects of Cost-Sharing in Healthcare', in *Effective Healthcare,* vol. 1 (1), 1983, pp. 47–57.

5 Stephen Birch, 'Increasing Patient Charges in the NHS: A Method of Privatising Primary Care', *Journal of Social Policy,* vol. 15, 1986, p. 163.

6 R. H. Brook et al, 'Does Free Care Improve Adults' Health? Results from a Randomised Controlled Trial', *New England Journal of Medicine,* 8 December 1983.

7 Joseph Newhouse and The Insurance Experiment Group, *Free For All: Lessons from the RAND Health Insurance Experiment,* 1993.

8 Ibid. p. 339.

9 Ibid. p. 351.

10 British Dental Association, *Fact File,* London, BDA, 1997.

11 Nick Bosanquet and Anna Zarzecka, 'Attitudes to Health Services 1983 to 1993', in Anthony Harrison (ed.), *Healthcare UK 1994/95,* 1995, p. 90.

12 Office of National Statistics, *Living in Britain 1995: General Household Survey,* London, The Stationery Office, 1997, Table 9.3.

13 Birch, 'Hypothesis', *Age and Ageing,* 1989, p. 136.

14 House of Commons Health Committee, *Fourth Report on Dental Services, Session 1992–93,* p. ix.

15 Office of National Statistics, *Living in Britain 1995: General Household Survey*, London, HMSO, 1997, Table 9.4.

16 House of Commons Health Committee, p. xi.

17 Office of National Statistics, *Living in Britain 1995*, 1997, Table 9.12.

18 House of Commons Health Committee, p. ix.

19 Department of Health, *Health Survey for England 1995,* London, The Stationery Office, 1997, p. 63.

20 Office of Health Economics, *Compendium of Health Statistics,* 1997, Table 4.102.

21 Royal National Institution for the Blind, *Losing Sight of Blindness,* London, RNIB, 1997, p. 4.

22 British Medical Association/Association of Optometrists, *Free Eye Examinations for the Over-65s: The Arguments in Favour,* London, BMA, 1995, p. 1.

23 Cited in Richard Wormald et al, 'Time to Look Again at Sight Tests: Those at Greatest Risk of Glaucoma are not the Most Likely to Attend for Sight Tests', *BMJ,* vol. 314, 1997, p. 245.

24 Royal National Institution for the Blind, 1997, p. 4.

25 D. A. H. Laidlaw et al, 'The Sight-Test Fee: Effect on Ophthalmology Referrals and Rate of Glaucoma Detection', *BMJ,* vol. 309, 1994, p. 635.

26 M. W. Tuck and R. P. Crick, 'Screening for Glaucoma: Why is the Disease Underdetected?', *Drugs and Ageing,* vol. 10(1), 1997, p. 2.

27 Wormald et al, 1997, p. 24.

28 Office of Health Economics, 1997, Table 4.45.

29 Ibid. Tables 4.27, 4.28.

30 British Medical Association, *NHS Prescription Charges,* London, BMA Parliamentary Brief, April 1997.

31 R.J. Lavers, 'Prescription Charges, the demand for prescriptions and morbidity', *Applied Economics,* vol. 21, 1989, p. 1050.

32 Bernie O'Brien, 'The Effect of Patient Charges on the Utilisation of Prescription Medicines', *Journal of Health Economics,* vol. 8, 1989, p. 124.

33 Mandy Ryan and Stephen Birch, 'Charging for Healthcare: Evidence

on the Utilisation of NHS Prescribed Drugs', *Social Science and Medicine,* vol. 33(6), 1991, p. 685.

34 David Hughes and Alistair McGuire, 'Patient Charges and the Utilisation of NHS Prescription Medicines: Some Estimates Using a Cointegration Procedure', *Health Economics,* vol. 4, 1995, p. 220.

35 Office of Health Economics, 1997, Table 4.27.

36 O'Brien, 1989, p. 127.

37 Birch, 'Increasing Patient Charges', *Journal of Social Policy*, 1986, pp. 163, 169–70.

38 Birch, 'Hypothesis', *Age and Ageing*, 1989, p. 136.

39 Antonio Giuffrida and David Torgerson, 'Should We Pay the Patient? Review of Financial Incentives to Enhance Patient Compliance', *BMJ,* vol. 315, 1997, p. 703.

40 Newhouse and The Insurance Experiment Group, 1993, p. 356.

41 The evidence is reviewed in Margaret Whitehead and Finn Diderichsen, 'International Evidence on Social Inequalities in Health, in Frances Drever and Margaret Whitehead (eds.), *Health Inequalities,* London, HMSO, 1997, pp. 62–64.

Chapter 9: Closing the Health Gap

1 British Medical Association, *Options for Funding Healthcare,* London, BMA, 1997, p. 8.

2 The following sections draw heavily – but not entirely consistently – on Bill New and Julian Le Grand, *Rationing in the NHS: Principles and Pragmatism,* 1996.

3 Henry Aaron, 'Thinking about Healthcare Finance: Some Propositions', in Organisation for Economic Co-operation and Development, *Healthcare Reforms – The Will to Change,* 1996, p. 56.

4 Paul Belien, 'What Can Europe's Healthcare Systems Tell Us About the Market's Role?', in William McArthur, Celia Ramsay and Michael Walker (eds.), *Healthy Incentives: Canadian Health Reform in an International Context,* 1996, p. 42–44.

5 William Hsiao, 'Marketisation – the Illusory Magic Pill', *Health Economics,* vol. 3, 1994, p. 354.

6 Ibid. p. 354.

7 Howard Glennerster, *Paying for Welfare – Towards 2000,* 1997, p. 144.

8   Hsiao, 1994, p. 355.

9   New and Le Grand, *Rationing in the NHS*, 1996, p. 48.

10 This discussion draws heavily on Victor Fuchs, *The Future of Health Policy*, 1993, pp. 51–64, and Deborah Baker, 'Poverty and Disease: A Postcard from the Edge', *Journal of the Royal Society of Medicine*, vol. 88, March 1995, pp. 127–29.

11 Secretary of State for Health, *Our Healthier Nation*, 1998, para. 1.11.

12 Ibid, para. 1.9.

13 Daniel Dorling, *Death in Britain: How Local Mortality Rates Have Changed 1950s–1990s*, 1997.

14 Frances Drever and Margaret Whitehead, *Health Inequalities*, 1997, p. 100.

15 Ibid. p. 100.

16 Baker, 1995, p. 128.

17 Ibid. p. 128.

17 Fuchs, 1993, p. 54.

19 Department of Health, *Health Survey for England 1995*, London, The Stationery Office, 1997, Table 9.17.

20 Dorling, 1997, p. 46.

21 Raymond Illsley and Deborah Baker, *Inequalities in Health: Adapting the Theory to Fit the Facts*, 1997.

22 Secretary of State for Health, *Our Healthier Nation*, 1998, para. 2.5.

23 Fuchs, 1993, p. 56.

24 Baker, 1995, p. 128.

25 Secretary of State for Health, *The Health of the Nation: A Strategy for Health in England*, 1992.

26 Anthony Harrison and Bill New, 'Health Policy Review', in Harrison and New (eds.), *Healthcare UK 1996/97: An Annual Review of Healthcare Policy*, 1997, p. 43.

27 Secretary of State for Health, *Our Healthier Nation*, 1998, Chap. 4.

28 Antonio Giuffrida and David Torgerson, 'Should We Pay the Patient? Review of Financial Incentives to Enhance Patient Compliance', *BMJ*, vol. 315, 20 September 1997, pp. 703–07.

Chapter 10: Prescription for Recovery

1   Department of Social Security, *Households Below Average Income*,

London, The Stationery Office, 1997, Table 8.5.

2 Office for National Statistics, *Family Spending 1996–97,* London, The Stationery Office, 1997, Table 1.1.

3 Office of Health Economics, *Compendium of Health Statistics,* 1997, Table 2.7.

4 Henley Centre, *Planning for Social Change 1998,* 1998.

5 Richard Saltman and Casten von Otter, 'Vouchers in Planned Markets', in Saltman and von Otter (eds), *Implementing Planned Markets in Healthcare,* 1995, pp. 146–47.

6 J. Atri, M. Falshaw, R. Gregg, J. Robson, R.Z. Omar and S. Dixon, 'Improving Uptake of Breast-Screening in Multiethnic Populations: A Randomised Controlled Trial Using Practice Reception Staff to Contact Non-Attenders', *BMJ,* vol. 315, 22 November 1997, pp. 1356–59.

7 Secretary of State for Health, *The New NHS: Modern, Dependable,* 1997, paras. 2.14, 2.18, 2.20.

8 Martin Powell, *Evaluating the National Health Service,* 1997, p. 147.

9 *NHS To Be Judged On Quality Not Just Quantity of Care,* Department of Health press notice 97/160, 9 July 1997.

10 Alain Enthoven, *Reflections on the Management of the National Health Service,* 1985, p. 13.

11 Secretaries of State for Health, Wales, Northern Ireland and Scotland, *Working for Patients,* 1989, paras 1.2, 1.7.

12 Rudolf Klein, *The New Politics of the NHS* 1995, pp. 192–93.

13 Nick Bosanquet and Stephen Pollard, *Ready for Treatment,* 1997, p.52.

14 Ibid. p. 54.

15 Roger Douglas, *Unfinished Business,* 1993, p. 222.

Select Bibliography

Henry Aaron and W. B. Schwartz, *The Painful Prescription: Rationing Hospital Care,* Washington DC, Brookings Institute, 1984.

Judy Allsop, *Health Policy and the NHS* (2nd edn), Harlow, Longman, 1995.

Audit Commission, *Improving Your Image: How to Manage Radiology Services More Effectively,* London, Audit Commission, 1995.

Audit Commission, *By Accident or Design: Improving A&E Services in England and Wales,* London, Audit Commission, 1996.

Audit Commission, *What the Doctor Ordered: A Study of GP Fundholders in England and Wales,* London, Audit Commission, 1996.

Audit Commission, *Goods for Your Health: Improving Supplies Management in NHS Trusts,* London, Audit Commission, 1996.

Deborah Baker, 'Poverty and Disease: A Postcard from the Edge', *Journal of the Royal Society of Medicine,* vol. 88, March 1995, pp. 127–29.

Correlli Barnett, *The Lost Victory: British Dreams, British Realities 1945–1950,* London, Macmillan, 1995.

Nicholas Barr, 'Economic Theory and the Welfare State: A Survey and Interpretation', *Journal of Economic Literature,* vol. 30, June 1992, pp. 741-803.

Will Bartlett, 'Quasi-markets and contracts: a markets and hierarchies perspective on NHS Reform', *Public Money,* vol. 11(3), 1991, pp. 53–61.

Paul Belien, 'What Can Europe's Healthcare Systems Tell Us About the Market's Role?', in William McArthur, Celia Ramsay and Michael Walker (eds.), *Healthy Incentives: Canadian Health Reform in an International Context,* Vancouver, Fraser Institute, 1996.

Göran Berleen, Clas Rehnberg and Gunnar Wennström, *The Reform of Healthcare in Sweden,* Stockholm, SIPRI, 1993.

Stephen Birch, 'Increasing Patient Charges in the NHS: A Method of Privatising Primary Care', *Journal of Social Policy* 1986, vol. 15.

Stephen Birch, 'Hypothesis: Charges to Patients Impair the Quality of Dental Care to Elderly People', *Age and Ageing,* vol. 18, 1989, pp. 136–40.

A. Blenkinsopp and C. Bradley, 'Over The Counter Drugs: Patients, Society and the Increase in Self-Medication', *BMJ,* vol. 312, 1996, pp. 629–32.

Nick Bosanquet, 'Improving Health', in Roger Jowell et al (eds.), *British Social Attitudes: The 11th Report,* Aldershot, Dartmouth, 1994.

Nick Bosanquet and Anna Zarzecka, 'Attitudes to Health Services 1983 to 1993', in Anthony Harrison (ed.), *Healthcare UK 1994/95,* London, King's Fund, 1995.

Nick Bosanquet and Stephen Pollard, *Ready for Treatment,* London, Social Market Foundation/Profile, 1997.

Sean Boyle and Richard Hamblin, *The Health Economy of London,* London, King's Fund, 1997.

Lindsay Brook, John Hall and Ian Preston, 'Public Spending and Taxation', in Roger Jowell et al (eds.), *British Social*

Attitudes – The 13th Report, Aldershot, Dartmouth, 1996.

Michael Calnan, Sarah Cant and Jonathan Gabe, *Going Private: Why People Pay For Their Healthcare,* Buckingham, Open University Press, 1993.

David Colin-Thomé, *Why Fundholding Should Stay*, London, Social Market Foundation, 1997.

Mia Defever, 'Long-Term Care: The Case of the Elderly', *Health Policy,* vol. 19, 1991, p. 8.

Daniel Dorling, *Death in Britain: How Local Mortality Rates Have Changed 1950s–1990s,* York, Joseph Rowntree Foundation, 1997.

Roger Douglas, *Unfinished Business,* Auckland, New Zealand, Random House, 1993.

Frances Drever and Margaret Whitehead (eds.), *Health Inequalities,* London, The Stationery Office, 1997.

Alan Earl-Slater, 'Privatising Medicines in the National Health Service', *Public Money and Management,* vol. 16, January–March 1996, pp. 39–44.

Efficiency Scrutiny Team, *Prescription Fraud: An Efficiency Scrutiny,* London, NHS Executive, 1997.

Alain Enthoven, *Reflections on the Management of the National Health Service,* London, Nuffield Provincial Hospitals Trust, 1985.

John Eversley and Charles Webster, 'Light on the Charge Brigade', *Health Service Journal,* 17 July 1997, pp. 26–28.

Stephen Frankel and R. West (eds.), *Rationing and Rationality in the National Health Service: The Persistence of Waiting Lists,* London, Macmillan, 1993.

Victor Fuchs, *The Future of Health Policy,* Cambridge, Mass., Harvard University Press, 1993.

Thomas Getzen, 'Population Ageing and the Growth of Health Expenditures', *Journal of Gerontology,* Social Sciences, vol. 47(3), 1992, pp. S98–104.

Antonio Giuffrida and David Torgerson, 'Should We Pay the Patient? Review of Financial Incentives to Enhance Patient Compliance', *BMJ,* vol. 315, 1997, pp. 703–07.

Howard Glennerster, *Paying for Welfare – Towards 2000* (3rd edn), Hemel Hempstead, Prentice Hall, 1997.

Howard Glennerster, Manos Matsaganis, Pat Owens and Stephanie Hancock, 'GP Fundholding: Wild Card or Winning Hand?', in Robinson and Le Grand (eds.), *Evaluating the NHS Reforms,* London, King's Fund 1993.

Sholom Glouberman (ed.), *Beyond Restructuring: A Collection of Papers from a King's Fund International Seminar,* London, King's Fund, 1996.

Nick Goodwin, 'GP Fundholding: a Review of the Evidence', in Anthony Harrison (ed.), *Healthcare UK 1995/96*, London, King's Fund, 1996.

Roy Griffiths, NHS *Management Inquiry,* London, Department of Health and Social Security, 1983.

Chris Ham, *Public, Private or Community: What Next for the NHS?,* London, Demos, 1997.

Chris Ham (ed.), *Healthcare Reform – Learning from International Experience,* Buckingham, Open University Press, 1997.

Anthony Harrison (ed.), *Healthcare UK 1994/95: An Annual Review of Healthcare Policy,* London, King's Fund, 1995.

Anthony Harrison (ed.), *Healthcare UK 1995/96: An Annual Review of Healthcare Policy,* London, King's Fund, 1996.

Anthony Harrison and Bill New (eds.), *Healthcare UK*

1996/97: An Annual Review of Healthcare Policy, London,
King's Fund, 1997.

Anthony Harrison and Sally Prentice, *Acute Futures,*
London, King's Fund, 1996.

Anthony Harrison, Jennifer Dixon, Bill New and Ken
Judge, 'Can the NHS Cope in Future?', *BMJ,* vol. 314,
1997, pp. 139–42.

Healthcare 2000, *UK Health and Healthcare Services:
Challenges and Policy Options,* London, Healthcare 2000,
1995.

Peter Hennessy, *Never Again: Britain 1945–1951,* London,
Vintage, 1992.

Frank Honigsbaum, Stefan Holmström and Johan Calltorp,
Making Choices for Healthcare, Abingdon, Radcliffe
Medical Press, 1997.

William Hsiao, 'Marketisation – the Illusory Magic Pill',
Health Economics, vol. 3, 1994, pp. 351–57.

Raymond Illsley and Deborah Baker, *Inequalities in Health:
Adapting the Theory to Fit the Facts,* Bath, University of
Bath, 1997.

Ken Judge and Michael Solomon, 'Public Opinion and the
National Health Service: Patterns and Perspectives in
Consumer Satisfaction', *Journal of Social Policy,* vol. 22(3),
July 1993, pp. 299–327.

Ken Judge, Jo-Ann Mulligan and Bill New, 'The NHS: New
prescriptions Needed?', in Roger Jowell et al (eds.),
British Social Attitudes – The 14th Report, Aldershot,
Ashgate, 1997.

Rudolf Klein, *The New Politics of the NHS* (3rd edn),
London, Longman, 1995.

Rudolf Klein, Patricia Day and Sharon Redmayne,
  *Managing Scarcity: Priority Setting and Rationing in the
  National Health Service,* Buckingham, Open University
  Press, 1996.
William Laing, *Laing's Review of Private Healthcare 1997,*
  London, Laing and Buisson, 1997.
Nigel Lawson, *The View from No. 11,* London, Bantam Press,
  1992.
Julian Le Grand, 'Evaluating the NHS Reforms', in Ray
  Robinson and Julian Le Grand (eds.), *Evaluating the NHS
  Reforms,* London, King's Fund, 1993.
Julian Le Grand and Will Bartlett, *Quasi-Markets and Social
  Policy,* London, Macmillan, 1995.
Alan Maynard, 'Can Competition Enhance Efficiency in
  Healthcare? Lessons from the Reform of the UK
  National Health Service', *Social Science and Medicine,* vol.
  39(10), 1994.
Alan Maynard and Gerald Richardson, *Over-The-Counter
  Medicines,* London, Social Market Foundation, 1996.
Ministry of Health, *A National Health Service,* Cmnd 6502,
  London, HMSO, 1944.
Elias Mossialos, 'Citizens' Views on Healthcare Systems in
  the 15 Member States of the European Union', *Health
  Economics,* vol. 6, 1997, pp. 109–16.
National Association of Health Authorities and Trusts,
  Health and the Economy, Birmingham, NAHAT, 1994.
Bill New and Julian Le Grand, *Rationing in the NHS:
  Principles and Pragmatism,* London, King's Fund, 1996.
Bill New and Nicholas Mays, 'Age, renal replacement
  therapy and rationing', in Anthony Harrison and Bill

New (eds.), *Healthcare UK 1996/97,* London, King's Fund, 1997.

Joseph Newhouse and The Insurance Experiment Group, *Free For All: Lessons from the RAND Health Insurance Experiment,* Cambridge, Mass., Harvard University Press, 1993.

Office of Health Economics, *Compendium of Health Statistics,* (10th edn), London, OHE, 1997.

Organisation for Economic Co-operation and Development, *The Reform of Healthcare: A Comparative Analysis of Seven OECD Countries,* Paris, OECD, 1992.

Organisation for Economic Co-operation and Development, *Healthcare Reforms – The Will to Change,* Paris, OECD, 1996.

Martin Powell, *Evaluating the National Health Service,* Buckingham, Open University Press, 1997.

Radical Statistics Health Group, *Facing the Figures: What Is Really happening to the National Health Service?,* London, Radical Statistics, 1987.

Radical Statistics Health Group, 'NHS Indicators of "Success": What do they Tell Us?', *BMJ,* vol. 310, 1995, pp. 1045–50.

Sharon Redmayne, *Small Steps, Big Goals: Purchasing Policies in the NHS,* Birmingham, National Association of Health Authorities and Trusts, 1996.

Sharon Redmayne, Rudolf Klein and Patricia Day, *Sharing Out Resources: Purchasing and Priority Setting in the NHS,* Birmingham, National Association of Health Authorities and Trusts, 1993.

Geoffrey Rivett, *From Cradle to Grave: Fifty Years of the NHS,*

London, King's Fund, 1998.

Ray Robinson, *New Directions in Health Economics,* Southampton, Institute for Health Policy Studies, 1995.

Ray Robinson and Julian Le Grand (eds.), *Evaluating the NHS Reforms,* London, King's Fund, 1994.

Royal Commission on the National Health Service, *Report,* Cmnd 7615, London, HMSO, 1979.

Richard Saltman and Casten von Otter (eds.), *Implementing Planned Markets in Healthcare,* Buckingham, Open University Press, 1995.

Secretary of State for Health, *The Patient's Charter,* London, HMSO, 1991.

Secretary of State for Health, *The Health of the Nation: A Strategy for Health in England*, Cm 1986, London, HMSO, 1992.

Secretary of State for Health, *The New NHS: Modern, Dependable,* Cm 3807, London, The Stationery Office, 1997.

Secretary of State for Health, *Our Healthier Nation,* Cm 3852, London, The Stationery Office, 1998.

Secretaries of State for Health, Wales, Northern Ireland and Scotland, *Working For Patients,* Cm 555, London, HMSO, 1989.

Nicholas Timmins, *Cash, Crisis and Cure,* London, The Independent, 1988.

Nicholas Timmins, *The Five Giants: A Biography of the Welfare State,* London, HarperCollins, 1995.

Wynand van de Ven, 'Effects of Cost-Sharing in Healthcare', in *Effective Healthcare*, vol. 1(1), 1983, pp. 47–57.

Charles Webster, *The Health Services Since the War Vol 1: Problems of Healthcare – The National Health Service Before 1957,* London, HMSO, 1988.

Sarah Wordsworth, Cam Donaldson and Anthony Scott, *Can We Afford the NHS?,* London, Institute for Public Policy Research, 1996.

John Yates, *Why Are We Waiting? An Analysis of Hospital Waiting Lists,* Oxford, OUP, 1987.